OTHER BOOKS BY MARSHALL AND PHYLLIS KLAUS

Bonding: Building the Foundations of Secure Attachment and Independence
(with John H. Kennell, M.D.)

Mothering the Mother:
How a Doula Can Help You Have a Shorter, Easier, and Healthier Birth
(with John H. Kennell, M.D.)

YOUR AMAZING NEWBORN

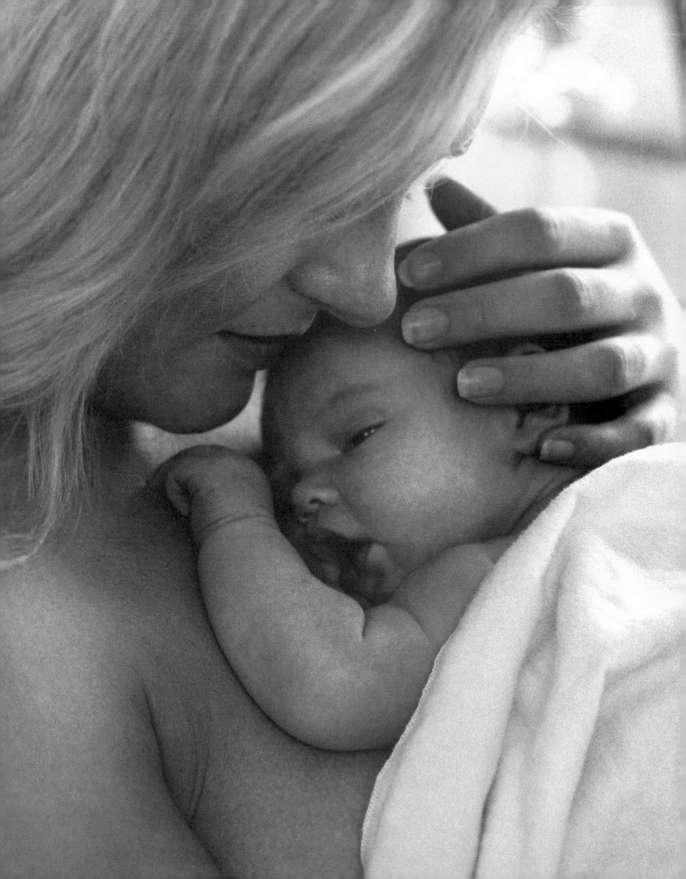

YOUR AMAZING NEWBORN

Marshall H. Klaus, M.D.
Phyllis H. Klaus, C.S.W., M.F.C.C.

A Merloyd Lawrence Book

PERSEUS BOOKS
Cambridge, Massachusetts

A CIP catalogue record for this book is available through the Library of Congress

ISBN 0-7382-0188-X

Cover design by Suzanne Heiser
Cover photographs by Jamie Bolane
Text design by Janis Owens
Set in 10.5-point Electra by Janis Owens

Perseus Books is a member of the Perseus Books Group.

6 7 8 9 10 RRD(HSB) 03 02 01
First paperback printing, December 1999

Perseus Books are available at special discounts for bulk purchases in the U.S. by corporations, institutions, and other organizations. For more information, please contact the Special Markets Department at HarperCollins Publishers, 10 East 53rd Street, New York, NY 10022, or call 1-212-207-7528.

Find us on the World Wide Web at http://www.perseusbooks.com

We dedicate this book with much love and appreciation to Susan;
David and Laura, Michael and Abigail; Alisa; Laura and David, Emily,
and Sharon; Sarah, John, Jocelyn, and Geoffrey—all wonderful children
and grandchildren from whom we have learned so much.

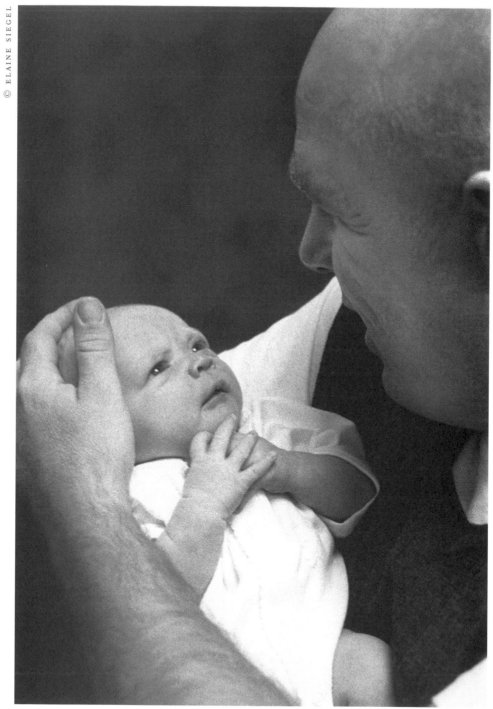

CONTENTS

PREFACE

This is an exciting time for those of us who enjoy baby and parent watching. Most maternity centers now make it possible for parents to become acquainted with their new infant at their own pace, even keeping their baby with them the entire time until they go home. There is also much more knowledge about what the baby, mother, and father bring to these early minutes and days of life. Not long ago, Swedish midwives discovered that infants, when dried and placed on their mother's abdomen after birth, have the ability after a short resting period to find their way to the mother's breast and latch on all by themselves. The search to learn how the baby might make this trip has led to interesting connections. For instance, we have inquired whether the baby's interest in light and dark contrasts and its preference for circles rather than squares might explain an attraction to the darkened areola of the nipple, the goal of the newborn's first short journey.

The human infant and mother evolved over 400,000 years in an environment different from today's. The body, the behavior, and the skills of both mother and infant have evolved to aid in their survival.

In this book we have brought together new and sensitive insights from many creative researchers, describing and photographing their findings about infants. When parents and other caregivers are able to read accurately and become attuned to their baby's responses and needs, they begin to feel more confident. A new appreciation of the baby brings a cascade of positive effects in the baby's social, physical, and mental development as well as in the adults' comfort with their caretaking efforts.

We previously observed that when we noticed a unique behavior in a particular infant for the first time, we suddenly began to see it in other infants. Often, this was an ability previously believed beyond the infant's capacity. When we first saw a one-day-old infant reaching and touching a parent's face, we began to see other infants with the same ability. When readers see photographs in this book of various kinds of behavior, they will then be able to spot them a bit more easily in their own infants.

However, we should caution readers that each baby has a mind of his own and may not want to carry out the behaviors at any particular time. In this early period, you may get a glimpse of any activity for only a few moments. Do not expect an infant to perform all the various antics. Additionally, some behaviors occur only when your infant is in the special state of quiet alertness. Nevertheless, these observations are intended to add to a parent's pleasure, to show

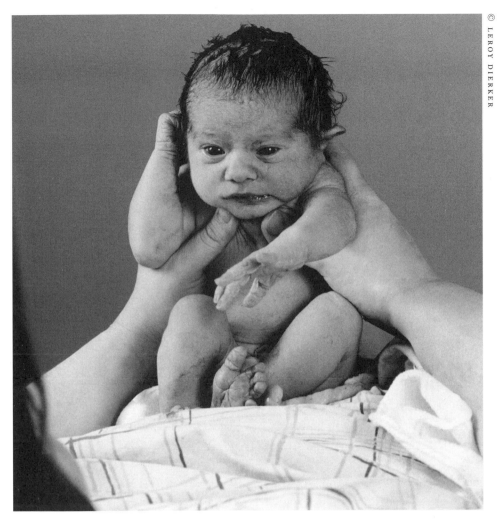

Thirty seconds old

what the changes in behavior might mean, and to help each reader discover the attributes of his or her own infant.

In our recent observations of a group of newborns and their parents shortly after birth, we informed several of the parents beforehand of newborns' ability to reach the breast on their own. Many of the mothers and fathers wanted their infants to attempt this journey. They held back from placing their babies on the breast, and let the infants achieve this on their own. We were pleased to witness how the accomplishment of this task changed the parents' view of their own baby. As one mother remarked, "I am

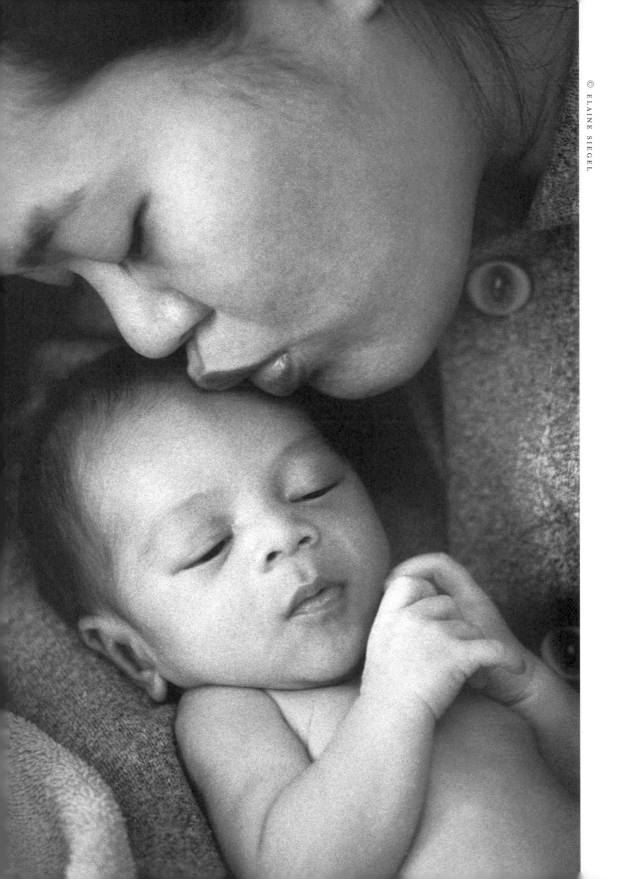

amazed at what he has inside of him. You know, this strength, vigor, determination, these are things you don't get later in life. I think I am pretty pleased to see so early what this little guy is made of."

We also hope that nurses, physicians, and educators involved in childbirth and newborn care will find the information in this book useful as they adapt and alter their caregiving practices to reflect what is now known about the abilities of the infant and their parents.

We appreciate the unique photographic talents and astute pictorial supervision of Elaine Siegel, who contributed so creatively in capturing the spontaneous nature of these young subjects. We additionally thank the other very talented photographers whose skills added greatly to the book as well as the expert and artistic digital image preparation of Bob Sekelsky.

We also benefited from many discussions with Anna-Berit Ransjo-Arvidson, Kyllike Christensson, Eva Nissen, Ann-Marie Widstrom, and Professor Kerstin Uvnäs-Moberg, talented Swedish

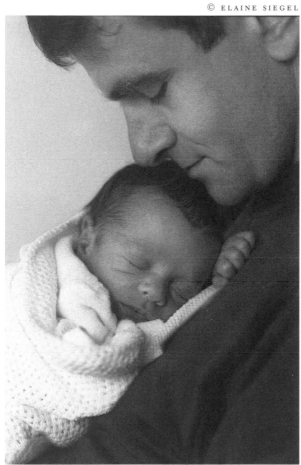

© ELAINE SIEGEL

researchers who first noted a number of the discoveries we describe. In addition, special thanks to Bonnie Petrauskas, Julia Freedman, and the Johnson & Johnson Company, who helped make it possible to develop a new film titled *The Amazing Talents of the Newborn*, which demonstrates many of the abilities we describe in this book. We are very fortunate to have a unique editor, Merloyd Lawrence, whose strong support and broad knowledge in this field has skillfully guided us in this project. Thanks also to our secretary, Nancy Pino.

Probably we have benefited most from the parents and the babies themselves who have taught us much and helped us better understand this early period in life. We fervently hope that in the beginning of the twenty-first century, medical caregivers will catch up to these many new discoveries and adjust their care practices to fit and to nurture the behavioral, emotional, and physiological processes built into newborns and their parents.

YOUR AMAZING NEWBORN

BEFORE BIRTH:
DAWNING AWARENESS

The world of the human fetus is alive with activity, with special rhythms, with movements that have purpose, with senses that are beginning to work—seeing, hearing, tasting, and feeling—and with complex responses to the emotions and actions of its mother. All this activity prepares babies not only for the huge changes ahead, but also, in the first minutes following birth, to interact with their parents.

Surprisingly, each fetus determines when it wants to be born. A small specific area of the brain sets in motion a series of events that will lead to the beginning of labor. Labor in turn stimulates babies in ways that prepare them to survive in the outside world. The mother and baby are on the journey together.

Early in pregnancy many parents start dreaming about their baby. What will the baby look like? Will it be a boy? a girl? The first visual evidence to fit into this dream is often an ultrasound picture. On the screen, parents first glimpse the tiny form, with its heart beating. At that moment, many

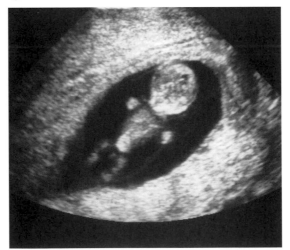

10 weeks
ALL FETAL PHOTOS CHAPTER 1 © JASON BIRNHOLZ

parents begin feeling attached to the baby. For others, this attachment will begin after feeling the baby move—the quickening—for still others, when they meet the baby for the first time, and for many others, in the first week of life. There is emotional as well as physical change in this early period of development.

Our notion of what life is like for the human fetus becomes clearer each year. Ultrasound images, magnetic resonance imagery, fiber optic and other innovative technologies, as well as careful observations of very premature infants who survived early delivery, have given us a glimpse of the fetus and its capacities to react, to perceive light and sound, to register sensations or sensory messages. We know much more about how intrauterine experience and activities rehearse and prepare the fetus for life outside the uterus.

Though ultrasound is probably safe, not everything about its effect is yet known. Most doctors recommend that it be used only when necessary. In practice, ultrasound is used mainly to estimate the age of the fetus by measuring the dimensions of its head. This calculation is most accurate when done between fifteen and thirty weeks of pregnancy. Ultrasound is also used to check for certain problems in development.

Through these various imaging techniques, we can follow the growth of the fetus from its beginning weeks of life. At twenty-three days the beating heart is the first movement that can be seen in the fetus. By means of an ultrasound image, we can see that a five-week-old fetus is capable of spontaneous movement.

At about four to five months of pregnancy, mothers begin to feel the fetus move, and fathers—when they rest their hands on the mother's abdomen—shortly after that. However, undetected motion has already been occurring for some time. By seven to eight weeks, the fetus can accomplish very simple movements of a single arm or leg joint, the wrist, elbow, or knee. At twelve weeks, the fetus can move all the joints of an arm or leg together. By thirteen or fourteen weeks, the arms may move with the legs, and sometimes the fetus can even be seen to hold its hands up. By nineteen weeks, the fetus can step, hold itself erect, and scoot itself forward by bracing against a hand.

Such abilities have been seen both in ultrasound images and in tiny premature babies. Motion itself is essential for the growth and development of the muscles and bones as well as for the stimulation of nerve-cell growth in the brain. By twenty weeks of age, the main cortical nerves in the brain are in place. An extension of the nerve cells in the brain actually grows into an arm or a leg. Motion helps this growth and, at the same time, creates new pathways for future nerves. This process permits children as they grow to develop very fine hand control, for example. The movements of arms and legs can be compared to the work of a shuttle in a loom that weaves through the warp of the fabric, adding a new row of thread to the cloth with each motion. If movement is prevented in any limb, the joint freezes, muscles and nerves wither, and the bone atrophies. Thus the movements felt by a pregnant parent are crucial for the baby's development.

In the floating and weightless environment of the amniotic sac, the fetus has a wide range of freedom to move, keeping the joints flexible. The rocking motions that the fetus experiences in utero may explain why, after birth, the newborn derives so much pleasure from being held and rocked.

As researchers have observed the fetus using ultrasound, they have noticed a variety of surprising behaviors. Yawning, swallowing, breathing, rooting, smiling, grimacing, sucking, grasping, stretching, curling, and unfolding appear to be practiced for long periods before they are necessary. This rehearsal, like the training of an athlete, helps make each motion more smooth and coordinated over time.

The activity and life of the fetus are governed by a series of internal clocks, each running on a different schedule. The heart beats around 140 times a minute. This rate has been seen to

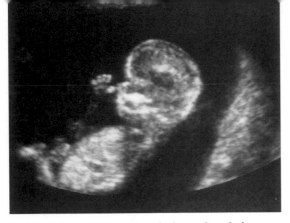

This 14-week-old fetus already has a hand close to its mouth.

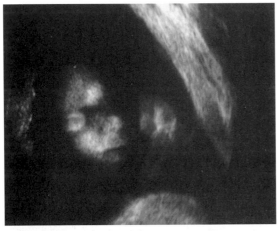

Facial features are clearly delineated at 18 weeks.

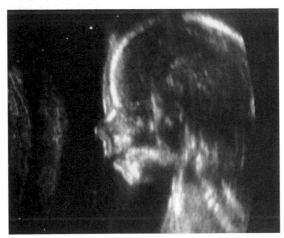

Is this 19-week-old fetus smiling?

change in response to noise, cigarette smoking by the mother, and even emotional stress in the mother. The timer controlling sleep and awake periods in the uterus is paced very slowly, changing once every thirty minutes. The timing of these sleep and awake states changes with the age of the fetus. Most of the clocks are located in the brain; however, the pacemaker for the fetal heart is part of the heart itself. These many clocks work simultaneously and produce overlapping rhythms in the fetus. Each baby has her own characteristic timetable and rhythm when born, and often mothers notice indications of these during pregnancy.

The environment of the womb is a symphony of sounds and vibrations. Minute microphones placed alongside the fetus at six to seven months have revealed that the volume of maternal sounds is slightly lower than that of a busy city street! The swishing of the mother's blood through her large blood vessels, her heartbeat, and her intestinal rumblings make up many of the sounds. The mother's voice also reaches the fetus, and, as we shall see in Chapter 5, the fetus can often distinguish its mother's voice from others.

In varying degrees, the fetus is sensitive to external noise and learns to tune out intrusive noise. Experiments with buzzers have demonstrated this ability to tune out, or habituate, as researchers call it. Such an ability shows a highly sophisticated level of development in the fetus.

Further evidence of fetal hearing comes from observing the fetus through ultrasound while it is responding to clicking sounds from outside the mother's abdomen. At twenty-eight weeks, an external clicking sound produces an immediate response of the eye. Eye blinks begin in some fetuses as early as twenty-six weeks, and all healthy fetuses blink by twenty-eight weeks. Researchers cannot yet tell how much of this blinking comes from the actual hearing of the click and how much is related to picking up the vibrations of the click with other sense organs. However, brain waves of very young premature infants show a definite response to pure sound as early as twenty-seven weeks of gestation. If you are ever concerned that your unborn baby is too quiet and not moving, try placing a small transistor radio on your abdomen and playing some music. You will immediately know all is well when it responds to the music by moving.

As parents have long noticed, fetuses display marked individual differences. Their levels of activity and responsiveness are, in part, related to later temperament, which we have learned from studies of identical twins is in large part genetically determined.

The mother's activities, physical movement, and feelings, however, have a strong influence on the behavior and physiological responses of the fetus. For example, if the mother consumes a large amount of sugar, which passes from her blood through the placenta into the fetus's circulation, the fetus may respond with increased activity. A prolonged, warm bath may make its body temperature rise slightly.

Even taste is developed long before delivery. Research with premature infants has shown that some taste receptors are developed between twenty-eight and thirty weeks. Young premature infants suck with extra vigor when given something sweet and make a face or grimace when given something tart.

The fetus's response to touch probably explains some of the movements the mother feels. When the soles of the feet touch something, the fetus will straighten its legs; and when its fingers come to its lips, it will suck on them. As early as six to eight weeks, if a fetus's hand or foot accidentally touches something in utero, the fingers or toes will curl; and by six months, the hand grasp is strong enough to actually support the fetus's own weight.

As we see in the ultrasound pictures, from the fourteenth to the thirty-sixth week the hands of the fetus are often in the vicinity of the face, touching and exploring the skin. Sometimes fetuses suck on their fingers and thumbs, per-

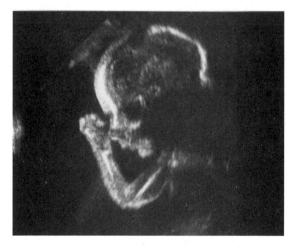

From the 14th to the 36th week, hands are often seen near the fetus's face. This fetus is 20 weeks old.

haps preparing the baby for sucking, soothing herself, and signaling her needs. This extensive early hand-to-face activity in the fetus may have other benefits. Learning to locate the face with the fingers before birth may help prepare the baby to imitate her parents' faces shortly after birth.

Sight develops several months before the pregnancy is full term. When a bright light is flashed on and off on the mother's abdomen, the fetus can be seen on an ultrasound to blink, but the blink occurs with a definite delay of one second, compared with the immediate blink in response to sound. Very premature infants are sometimes born with their eyelids still fused, but they do make a blinking motion at the flash of a bright light. Since light can be transmitted through the thin wall of a uterus and abdominal wall of the mother, the fetus probably experiences night and day. Premature babies who have spent only thirty to thirty-one weeks in the uterus already have visual preferences. When shown thick and thin stripes, they demonstrate that they prefer to look at thick stripes. These preferences keep changing, and by thirty-five to thirty-six weeks, they like to look at different kinds of shapes.

The fetus and mother become acquainted with each other in many ways, and mothers are the translators of many of these responses to their partners, who can only imagine what these activities are like. Some fathers enjoy visualizing what the baby is like, putting their hands on the mother's belly and sending their own loving messages to their child. Making an effort to con-

nect with their infant has helped many fathers feel more like participants rather than merely onlookers in this period.

Changing emotions for mother and father are common during this time. Sharing these feelings, communicating with each other, and endeavoring to understand the incredibly complex development going on in their child-to-be is part of the path to becoming parents. Fetal development, like later growth, is part nature, part nurture. Some of the movements and responses are innate, whereas others are stimulated or affected by the external environment. One can think of the DNA code in every cell in the infant's body as a composer's musical score; the manner in which the musicians play, how they interpret that score, resembles the environmental influences on how the code is expressed.

Brain activity has been seen as early as six weeks. At seven weeks, nerve cells in the brain have become connected along primitive nerve paths. Movements change from simple twitching to startles to complex actions. From sound and changing breathing patterns, the fetus forms a memory of its mother's and father's voices and develops distinct sleep and awake cycles.

Observations of pregnant women add continually to those of researchers. Many women have reported that the fetus responds by a change of activity to their emotions. Sometimes when mothers relax, the baby in the uterus appears to become more active. Is the mother just noticing her fetus more, or are chemical mediators actu-

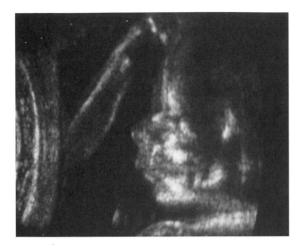

21 weeks

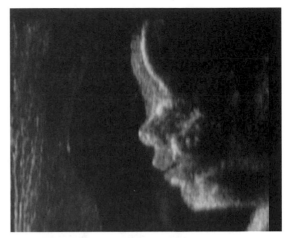

Contented expression at 30 weeks

ally being sent to the fetus when she takes a nice relaxing breath and imagines herself in a peaceful scene?

Mothers sometimes talk about a special way they communicate with their unborn baby. Often, in a quiet state of reverie, they visualize the infant to-be, or send the baby a message, or ask the baby a question, or sometimes sense a response from the baby.

In contrast, fetuses of women with chronic stress have fast heart rates and are very active. Women exposed to very high noise levels have been shown to risk premature delivery, apart from the effects of noise on the fetus mentioned earlier. By some complicated process, the fetus can be affected by biochemical changes caused by the mother's emotional experiences. Consequently, the mother and her baby are engaged in a dialogue long before the baby's birth. Her activity level and emotional state interlock with the unborn baby's characteristic cycles. As she adjusts to the rhythms of this new life within her, the fetus, in turn, is already experiencing the tempo of her life, and through her, that of its father and other members of its family.

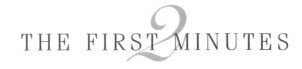

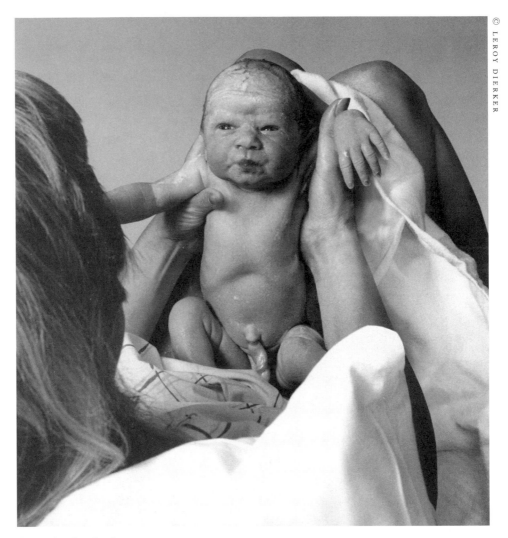

Seconds after birth

The first minutes of their baby's life are for parents an exciting, awesome, exhilarating, and exhausting experience. In these moments, all their dreams, hopes, and plans come together. After birth, the newborn is thoroughly dried with warm towels so as not to lose heat, and once it is clear that he has good color and is active and normal (usually within one to five minutes), he goes to his mother. Meanwhile, parents are yearning to know who their baby is, to see and hear and touch him, to make absolutely sure that the baby is normal and healthy. At this time, the warm and dry infant is placed between the mother's breasts or on her abdomen or right next to her as the family rests together for the next stage.

When newborns are kept close to their mother's body or on their mother, they apparently feel safe, and the transition from life in the womb to existence outside the uterus is made much easier for them. The newborn also recognizes his mother's voice and smell, and her body warms his. In this way the infant can experience sensations somewhat similar to what he felt during the last several weeks of uterine life.

When full-term infants are skin to skin with their mother, on her abdomen, chest, or in her arms, they very seldom cry during the first ninety minutes of life. However, when placed in a nearby bassinet, wrapped thoroughly, they cry about twenty to forty seconds during every five-minute period for the next ninety minutes. Newborns are already perceptive enough to know the difference between a bassinet and their mother!

A thoroughly dried infant placed on his

A few hours old

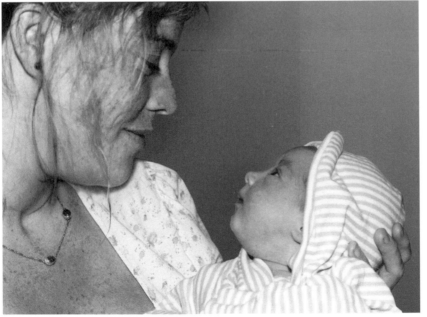

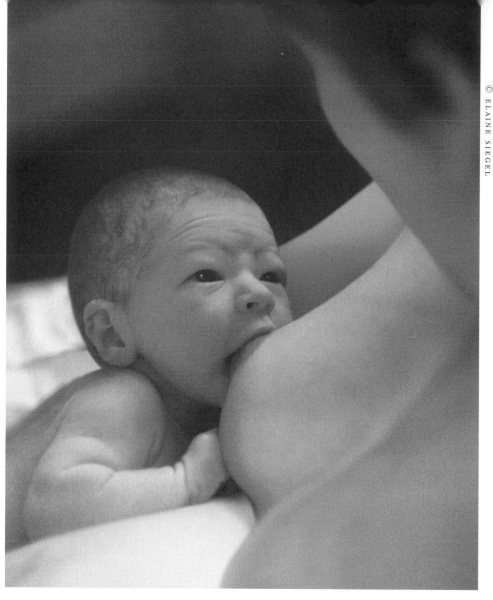

Less than one hour after birth, a newborn gazes at his mother.

mother's chest will warm up faster and in a healthier way than if placed in a bassinet fully covered with blankets. The mother will heat the baby to exactly the right temperature. Experience has shown that the mother's chest will even heat a chilled baby more quickly than will an incubator.

Many people believed in the past, and many believe even today, that the newborn needs help to begin to nurse. So, often, immediately after birth the baby's lips are placed near or on the mother's nipple. In that situation, some babies do start to suckle, but the majority just lick the nipple or peer up at the mother. They appear to be much more interested in the mother's face, especially in her eyes, even though the nipple is right next to their lips.

One of the most exciting observations made in our era is the discovery that the newborn has the ability to find his mother's breast all on his own and decide for himself when to take his first feeding. In order not to remove the taste and smell of the mother's amniotic fluid, it is necessary to delay washing the baby's hands. The baby uses the taste and smell of the amniotic fluid on his hands to make a connection with a certain oily substance on the nipple related to the amniotic fluid.

The infant usually begins with a time of rest and quiet alertness, during which he rarely cries and appears to take great pleasure in looking at his mother's face. Around thirty to forty minutes after birth, the newborn begins making mouthing movements, sometimes with lip smacking, and shortly after, saliva begins to pour down onto his chin. When placed on the mother's abdomen, babies maneuver in their own ways to reach the nipple. They often use stepping motions of their legs to move ahead, while to move horizontally toward the nipple, they use small push-ups, lowering one arm first in the direction they wish to go. These efforts are interspersed with short rest periods. Sometimes babies change direction in midstream. These actions take effort and time. Parents find patience well worthwhile as they wait and observe their infant on his first journey.

In the photos, one newborn is seen successfully navigating his own way. At ten minutes of age he first begins to move toward the left breast, but five minutes later he is back in the midline. Notice the repeated mouthing and sucking of the hands and fingers so commonly observed. Then, with a series of push-ups and rest periods, he makes his way to the left breast completely on his own, placing his lips on the areola of the breast. He now begins to suckle effectively and closely observes his mother's face. (Suckling on the areola prevents injury to the nipple itself, and babies who do this naturally will nurse for a longer period of time and injure or irritate the nipple less often.)

This sequence is helpful to the mother as well, since the massage of the breast induces a large oxytocin surge into her bloodstream, which helps contract the uterus, expelling the placenta, and closes off many blood vessels in the uterus, thus reducing bleeding. This stimulation and suckling also helps in the manufacture of prolactin, a hormone that stimulates milk production, and the suckling enhances the closeness and new bond between mother and baby. Mother and baby appear to be carefully adapted for these first moments together. Millions of years ago this adaptation served to save the mother's life and thereby that of her baby. Today we still marvel at a remarkable process!

We can also wonder whether the infant's visual interest in dark and light contrasts and preference for circles rather than squares fits together with the special interest the baby has at this time for the darkened circular appearance of the areola at the time of birth.

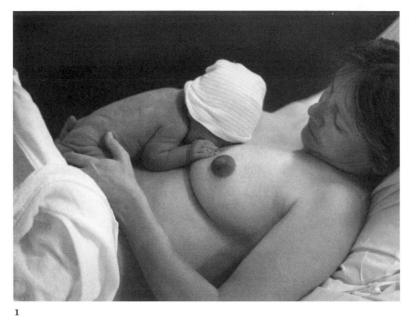

1 *Ten minutes after birth, this baby was placed between his mother's breasts.*

1

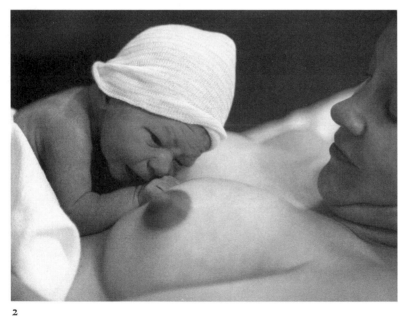

2 *After a few minutes he begins to maneuver, moving with small push-ups, first toward his mother's left breast.*

PHOTO SERIES
© ELAINE SIEGEL

2

3, 4 *He frequently stops to rest and suck on his fist and fingers.*

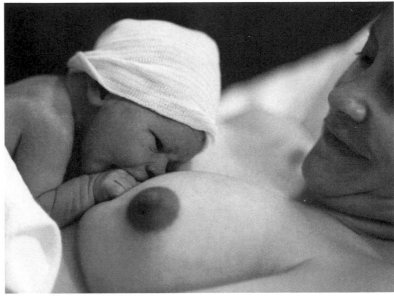

3

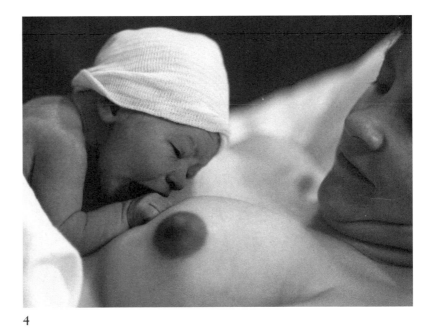

4

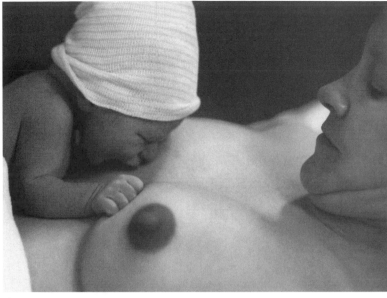

5 , **6** *With push-ups, he moves toward the right breast at 30 minutes.*

5

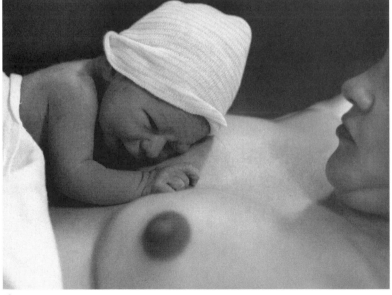

6

7 *Mother and infant gaze at each other.*

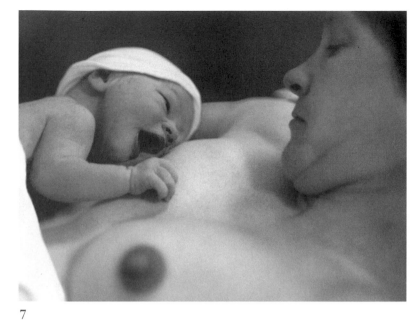

7

8 *Familiar with the taste and smell of amniotic fluid, he continues to suck on his unwashed hand and soon he moves to a similar smell emanating from the unwashed breast.*

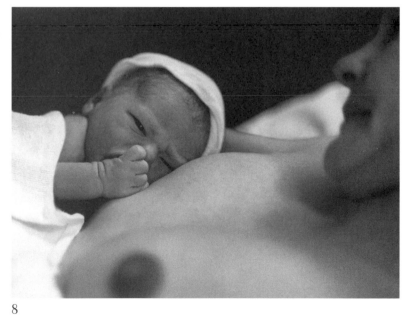

8

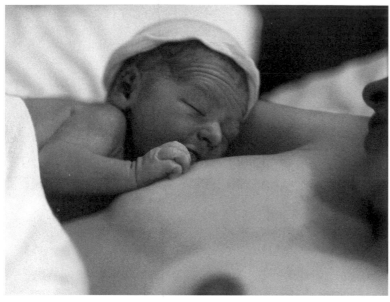

9, 10 *The baby begins to mouth the nipple, probably raising the mother's oxytocin levels.*

9

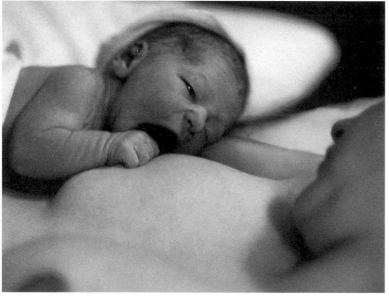

10

11, 12 The baby is readying
himself for a good placement
on the areola, opening his
mouth widely.

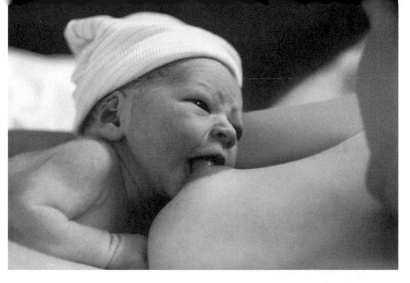

11

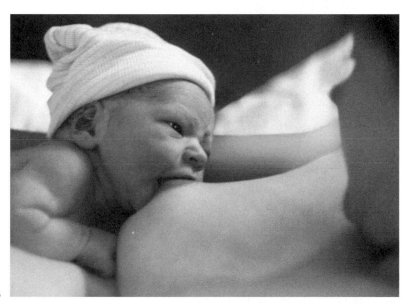

12

13 Sucking on the breast
while mother and infant look
at each other at around 50
minutes

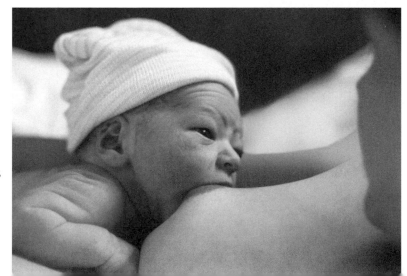

13

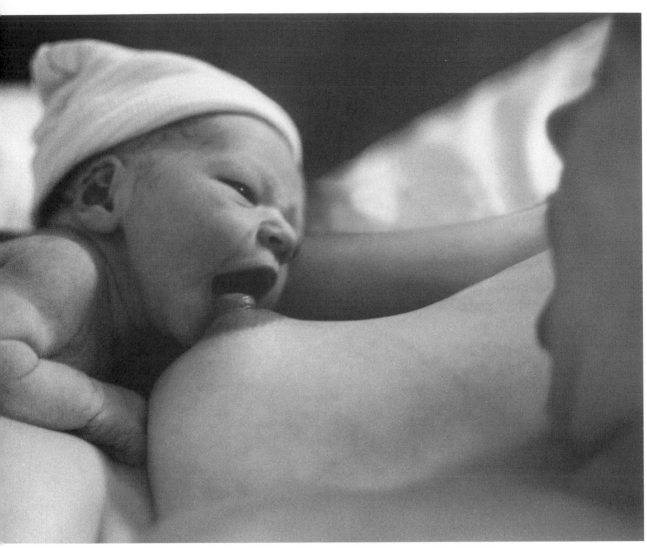

14 *Mother and infant both with their mouths wide open. Who is imitating whom?*

Many parents want this time right after birth kept sacred, for themselves and their baby. There is little that compares with the extraordinary sight of a baby only minutes old resting for a period, then quietly mouthing and licking his hands, and after a time moving to the breast and the nipple by a series of short push-ups, and beginning to suckle. Parents have urged hospitals to allow them to have this time without interruption. It is a significant and moving experience that they will always remember.

To allow this first intimate encounter, we strongly urge that the injection of vitamin K, application of eye ointment, washing, and any measuring of the infant's weight, height, and head circumference be delayed for at least an hour. Over 95 percent of all full-term infants are normal at birth. In a few moments they can be easily evaluated to assure that they are healthy. They can then after thorough drying be safely placed on their mother's chest if their parents wish.

This precious time for the mother, father, and baby must be protected. The family needs a quiet, softly lit room without much extraneous activity and with only a small number of people present. Mothers report feeling lonely and empty when relatives and hospital caregivers are engaged with the baby in a corner heat table and they are left alone. At a time when a mother desperately wants her baby close, if her desires are not respected she can feel isolated and abandoned. For many months during pregnancy a mother dreams of having her newborn in her own arms after the birth, and a period of time is needed to make an internal mental shift from the imagined or hoped-for baby to the real baby.

For mothers and fathers who decide to put their baby next to the mother right after birth rather than on the mother's chest or abdomen, it is good to know that the baby can feel close to the mother through the senses of smell and hearing and can begin to link up his mother's face with the voice already familiar from life in the womb. When the baby is placed next to the mother in this position, we recommend covering the baby with a shirt and diaper or a blanket, because he will not receive adequate heat from the mother's body and delivery rooms are often cold.

When trying to decide when to offer the first breast-feeding, parents can wait for the baby's signal. They can watch for mouthing movements, beginning with some lip smacking, and a flow of saliva, which do not usually occur for many minutes. When placed at the breast, or when the baby reaches the breast on his own, he opens his mouth wide, placing the lips and tongue in exactly the correct position. After several tries he generally latches onto the areola, the brown portion of the nipple. The odor of the nipple appears to guide a newborn to the breast. If the right breast is washed with soap and water, the infant will crawl to the left breast, and vice versa. If both breasts are washed, the infant will go to the breast that has been rubbed with the amniotic fluid of the mother. The special attraction of the newborn to the odor of his mother's amniotic fluid may reflect the time in

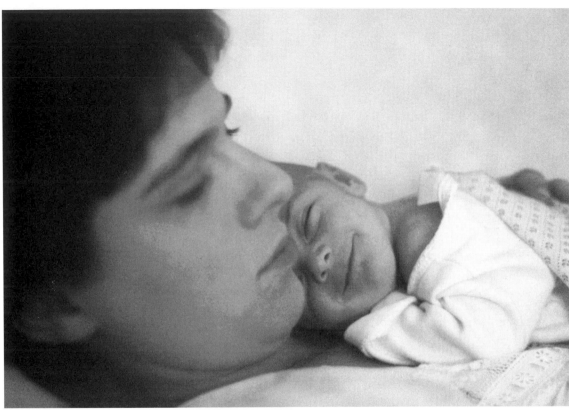

Is he smiling because he recognizes his mother's smell and voice, and feels the comfort of her warmth and touch?

utero when as a fetus, he swallowed the liquid. It appears that amniotic fluid contains a substance that is similar to some secretion of the breast, though not the milk. Amniotic fluid on the infant's hands probably also explains part of the interest in sucking the hands and fingers seen in the photographs. This early hand sucking behavior is markedly reduced when the infant is bathed before the crawl. With all these innate programs, it seems as if the infant comes into life carrying a small computer chip with these instructions.

In cultures in which customs of modesty prevail, mothers may feel more comfortable covered up. When a very light towel, sheet, or thin blanket covers both mother and infant, the baby can still easily maneuver toward the nipple in his own time. We heard from one mother from the Middle East, who had delivered in the Midwest of the United States. She was resting after the birth, the baby on her chest, both of them lightly covered, when all of a sudden she felt her baby attach herself to the nipple and begin sucking vigorously. The mother announced with great surprise and pleasure to the caregiver and her husband what had just occurred. She was delighted at her little girl's built-in talents.

At a moment such as childbirth we come full circle to our biological origins, realizing how infant survival may have depended on the innate capacity and energy of newborns to find the mother's breast. Many separate abilities enable a baby to do this. Stepping reflexes help the newborn push against his mother's abdomen to propel him toward the breast. Pressure of the infant's feet on the abdomen may also help in the expulsion of the placenta and in reducing uterine bleeding. The ability to move his hand in a reaching motion enables the baby to claim the nipple. Taste, smell, and vision all help the newborn detect and find the breast. Muscular strength in neck, shoulders, and arms helps newborns bob their heads and do small push-ups to inch forward and side to side. This whole scenario may take place in a matter of minutes, or it may take place within thirty to sixty minutes, but it is all within the capacity of the newborn. It is exciting to realize that our young, like other baby mammals, know how to find their mother's breast.

When the mother and infant are resting skin to skin and gazing eye to eye, they begin to learn about each other on many different levels. For the mother, the first minutes and hours after birth are a time when she's uniquely open emotionally to respond to her baby and to begin the new relationship. As parents recognize the special characteristics of their particular baby, they can more easily sense the baby's needs, and their ability and confidence to take care of their baby are enhanced. At the same time, as we will see in the next chapter, the newborn is in a uniquely alert state, ready to take in his family and his world.

WAKING TO ${3}$ THE WORLD

Something very special occurs within the first hour after birth. If the environment is quiet, the birthing without complications, the lights lowered, the handling diminished, newborn infants—aside from all the physiological adaptations they must make—begin in a uniquely human way to take in their new world.

One of the newborn's first responses is to move into a quiet but alert state of consciousness. In this state, the baby is still; her body molds to yours; her hands touch your skin; her eyes open wide and are bright and shiny. She looks directly at you.

This special alert state, this innate ability to communicate, may prepare the way for the future attachment between the newborn and those who care for her. The intensity and appealing power of this little bud of humanity meeting the world for the first time are all but irresistible.

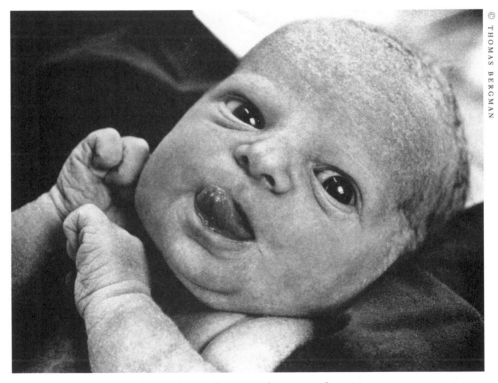

© THOMAS BERGMAN

Six minutes old, this infant girl is in the quiet alert state of consciousness.

Our understanding of the varied states of consciousness of the newborn began with the work of a child psychiatrist Peter Wolff, a psychologist Heinz Prechtl, and a pediatrician, T. Berry Brazelton. These researchers documented every aspect of newborn behavior: grimaces, hiccups, sneezes, tremors, and twitches. They noted arm and leg motion as well as breathing and sucking activity. They recorded minute eye and eyelid movements. In short, they documented any and all reflexes and responses to the environment. They found that seemingly random and unrelated activities actually fell into behavioral groups that made surprising sense. They classified these patterns into six different states of consciousness according to the infant's degree of wakefulness or sleep. By closely observing their own baby, parents can soon learn to recognize these states: the two sleep states, quiet sleep and active sleep; the three awake states, quiet alert, active alert, and crying; and drowsiness, a transition between sleep and wakefulness.

Each of these six states is accompanied by quite specific and individual behaviors. We do not understand how the brain produces the distinctions, but we do recognize that for the human infant there are six ways of being or acting in the world.

In the quiet alert state, which is very similar to the conscious attention we see in our friends when they are listening closely to us, babies rarely move. Their eyes are wide open, bright and shiny. In this state, newborns are especially fun to play with. They can follow a red ball,

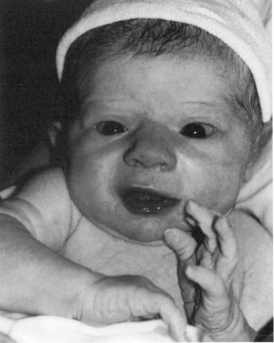

Minutes after birth, this infant is in the quiet alert state.

gaze at a face, turn to a voice, and they may even imitate a parent's expression.

Right after birth, within the first hour of life, normal infants have a prolonged period of quiet alertness, averaging forty minutes, during which they look directly at their mother's and father's faces and eyes and can respond to voices. It is as though newborns had rehearsed the perfect approach to the first meeting with their parents. (This may in fact be so; sleeping and waking states begin long before birth, as we saw in Chapter 1.) If the baby remains in close contact with her mother in the first hour of life, she will remain in the quiet alert state longer and cry

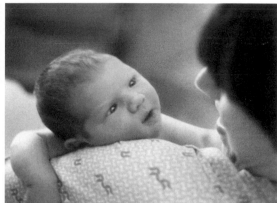

Newborn and his mother enjoying each other

hardly at all. Thus, the baby's state is already dependent on the care of those around her. In the quiet alert state, motor activity is suppressed and all the baby's energy seems to be channeled into seeing and hearing. Such alertness allows newborns to take in much of their surroundings and to respond and adapt to the environment.

During the first week of life, the normal baby spends about 10 percent of any twenty-four-hour day in this exciting and receptive state. After the first hour and a half of life, there is usually not such a prolonged period of the quiet alert state. The baby may be in this state for only short periods, especially around feeding. A majority of the exciting newborn talents that we discuss throughout this book can be observed only in the quiet alert state.

During the active alert state, the baby is very different. There is frequent movement, her eyes look about, sometimes around the room, and she makes small sounds. This state appears before eating or when the baby is fussy.

Although the baby does not move continuously, episodes of movement occur with a special rhythm. About every one to two minutes, the baby will move her arms, legs, body, or face. These movements may serve an adaptive purpose. Some scientists believe that they convey clues to parents about what their baby needs or that they promote a natural interaction between parent and baby. Similar bursts of movement, which may be regulated by some sort of internal clock within the baby's brain, have also been detected in the fetus, through sensitive measuring devices placed on the mother's abdomen late in pregnancy. In this active alert state the baby's attention is drawn to many different parts of the room. She shows interest in objects, but pays little attention to faces. As the parents get to know their baby, it is helpful for them to recognize the different activities and ways of being in these two awake states. The first evidence of natural curiosity emerges as the infant searches to understand her world.

The crying state, which is one obvious way for infants to communicate, occurs when the baby is hungry, uncomfortable, or lonely. An infant's eyes may be open or tightly closed when crying, the face is contorted and red, and the arms and legs move vigorously. Many parents know that they can change babies' crying states by picking them up, soothing them, and putting them to the shoulder, as shown here. Parents who pick up their crying infants are giving them an opportunity not only to be quietly awake, but also to learn about their world by scanning the room. Originally, researchers thought it was the

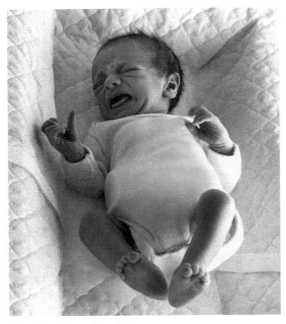

Newborn in crying state

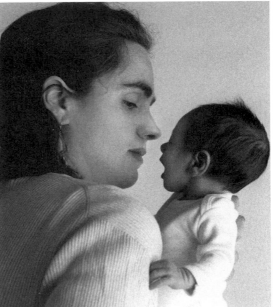

Mother picks him up.

upright position that soothed the baby. However, it turns out that it is the movement toward that position, rather than the position itself, that puts the baby into the quiet alert state. If the parent picks up the infant within a minute and a half of the onset of crying, she will promptly stop.

The baby's different signals and different qualities of crying are the language she speaks. Babies may also shut down or turn away when overstimulated. They may attempt to comfort themselves in many ways, putting fist or fingers in their mouths, continuing to cry, or eventually falling asleep. Parents who respond to the requests or signals of the infant teach her that her needs will be met and the world is good and caring.

Parents need to be detectives to unravel the many signals and cries of their infant. Sometimes it takes many tries to figure it out. Some mothers find that within about ten days they can pick up the hunger signal, the discomfort cry, and the sleepy cue, but sometimes other complaints are less easily understood. Holding the baby close, murmuring soothing words, and especially keeping oneself calm can be helpful in reading the baby's signals.

Infants cannot easily soothe themselves when under stress. They actually release stress hormones through tears and obvious distress, but do not always have the capacity to calm or completely relax themselves back to a normal, nonstressed state. They need human touch, holding, and a soothing voice. In some complex way

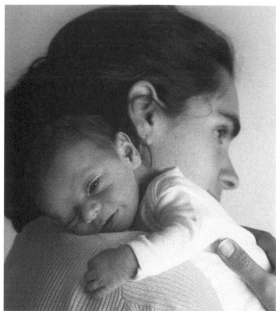

He becomes quiet and alert.

this caring touch causes the stress to lessen and, with their parents' help, babies eventually learn to calm themselves. When a baby is in much distress and crying, it is important to soothe and hold her, not only so that she will quiet down, but, more important, so that she learns that her parent is there, that she is safe, and that she can relax.

The drowsy state usually occurs while the baby is waking up or falling asleep. The baby may continue to move, sometimes smiling, frowning, or pursing her lips. Her eyes can have a dull, glazed appearance and usually do not focus. The eyelids are droopy, and just before closing, the eyes may roll upward. On awakening, the baby may make stretching movements, first on one side and then on the other.

During the newborn period, an infant sleeps

Father and baby can now enjoy each other.

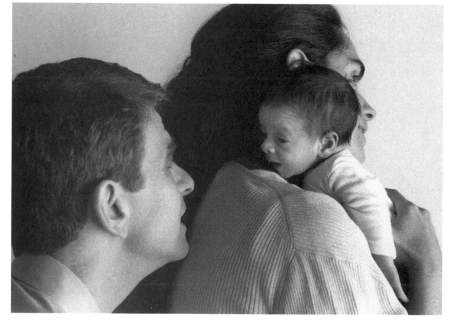

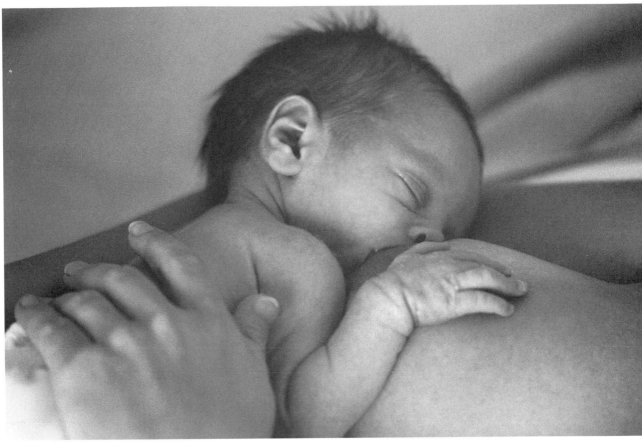

Newborn in deep sleep on mother's breast

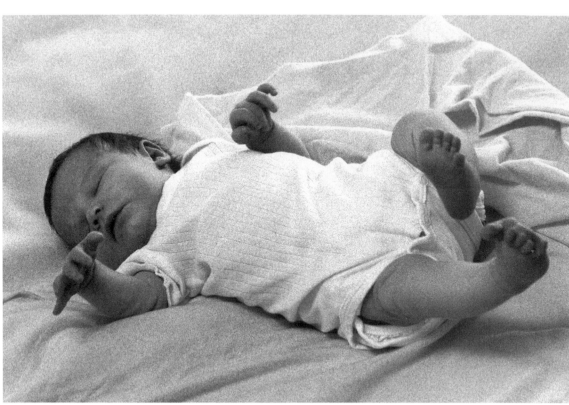

Busy arms and legs in active sleep

most of the time—about 90 percent of the day or night—and will often fall asleep right at the breast. Half this sleep time is spent in quiet sleep, the other half in active sleep. These two states alternate about every thirty minutes during sleep.

In quiet sleep, the baby's face is relaxed and the eyelids are closed and still. There are no body movements except rare startles and extremely fine mouth movements. In this state, babies are at full rest; breathing is very regular because they are taking in the same amount of air with each breath. However, in all states,

babies take a deep sigh every several minutes, which allows the lungs to be properly filled with just the right amount of air.

In active sleep, an infant's eyes are usually closed, but occasionally they will flutter from closed to open. One can often see the eyes move under the lids. Eye motion or stillness accompanying these two sleep states has even been observed in the fetus by means of ultrasound. The term *rapid eye movement*, or REM, sleep refers to the eye movements observed during this type of restless sleep.

In active sleep, occasional body activity

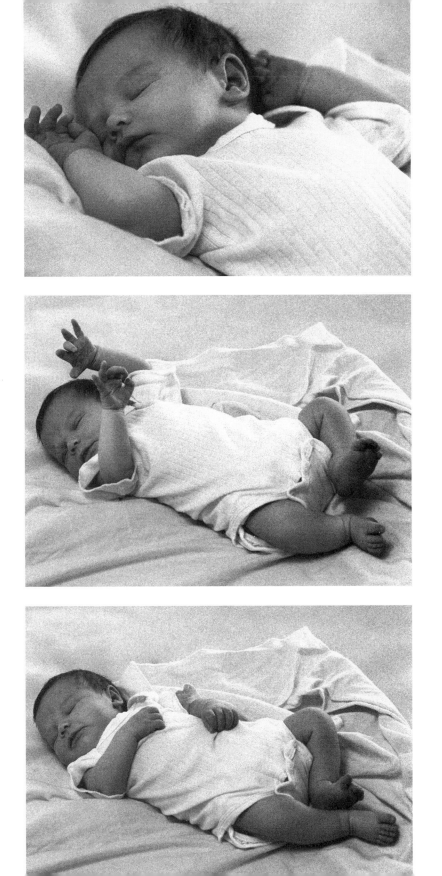

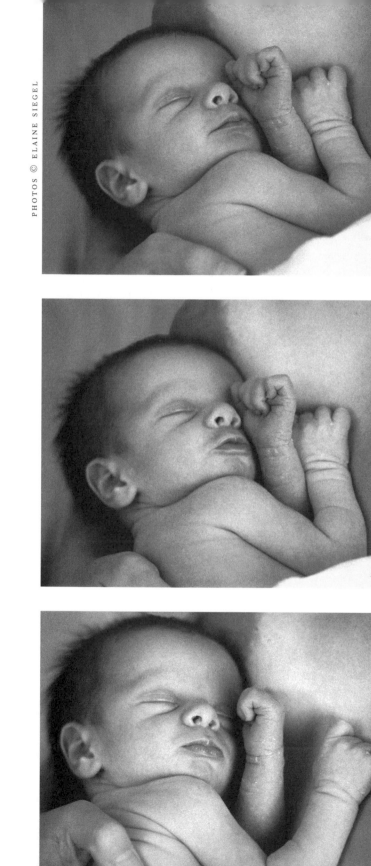

Changing expression in active sleep

ranges from movement of the arms and legs to stirring of the entire body. Breathing is not regular and can be slightly faster than it is in quiet sleep. While they remain asleep, infants in this state often make funny faces—grimaces, smiles, frowns—and may display chewing movements or bursts of sucking. When babies wake, they usually have been in active rather than quiet sleep. Adults dream while in REM sleep; no one knows whether infants also dream in this particular sleep state.

Babies in active sleep have occasionally been observed to move from one side of the crib to the other. They tend to gravitate toward an edge, especially toward a soft object. In one study, infants preferred to lie close to a breathing toy bear rather than a nonbreathing toy bear. Mothers have commented on how close their baby stays to them when in bed together after a feeding or while sleeping. In sleep, do babies remember the close connection with the walls of the womb, the sounds of their mother's heartbeat, and her internal rhythms? One father laughingly recalled that whenever his wife moved in the bed, the baby moved with her. He soon found himself scrunched over to one side, while the sleeping pair of mother and infant was very comfortable.

From these classifications of infant states of consciousness and observations of newborn babies' behavior, T. Berry Brazelton developed the very valuable Neonatal Behavioral Assessment Scale which has had a major influence in making both care givers and parents aware of the newborn's innate abilities.

Parents not only can get to know their infant by recognizing the different states and realizing when they occur and what the expected responses are in each, but also can provide most sensitively for her needs. For instance, when a baby is whimpering slightly and stirring in active sleep, a parent who is aware that this occurs in thirty-minute cycles will not rush to feed or change the baby unless this gentle activity turns into the active awake state and crying starts. Once parents understand and recognize the six patterns of newborn behavior, the mysterious, shifting world of the infant begins to make much more sense.

NEWBORN SIGHT

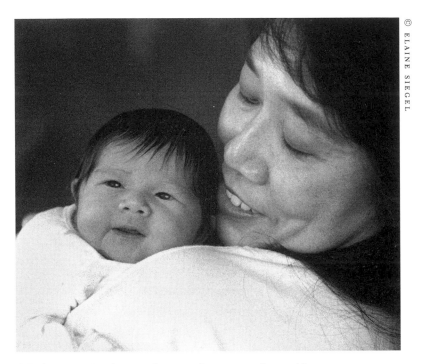

Mother enjoying her newborn as she surveys the world

The newborn's ability to see, once doubted, has been confirmed and demonstrated by decades of interesting experiments and observations. In 1996, T. G. R. Bower, who has spent his career studying newborns, found, with his colleagues, that full-term newborns can recognize their own mother's face as early as four hours after birth. To make this determination the researchers set up an ingenious experiment. Newborns were positioned in front of a video screen on which were flashed pairs of women's faces, including their mother's face. The infants were given pacifiers to suck, connected to a control on the screen. If a newborn sucked one way, one woman would appear; if he sucked another way, his mother would appear. After a period of watching and sucking, the newborns tended more often to suck in a way that brought their own mother's face onto the screen.

The ability of a newborn to recognize and distinguish different patterns was discovered in the 1960s by Dr. Robert Fantz. His studies of newborn visual fixation led psychologists and the medical profession to recognize and explore the amazing visual capacities of the newborn.

Dr. Fantz's procedure was based on the fact that a picture that is being looked at, or fixated, is reflected from the cornea of the eye over the pupil. When the reflection of the picture is seen on the surface of the pupil (the black portion within the center of the eye), the picture is aligned in such a way that it falls on the center of the retina (a recording device within the eye that relays the visual image to the brain).

In his experiments, an infant who had reached a quiet alert state was placed under a hood where he was shown two pictures. A peephole between the two pictures enabled an observer to discover easily what the baby was looking at by watching the baby's pupils.

In the illustration of the eye shown here, two patterns—a checkerboard and a plain white square—are reflected on the surface of the eye.

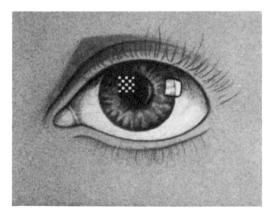

The infant is looking at a checkerboard pattern, since the checkerboard pattern can be seen directly over the pupil.

Since the checkerboard is directly over the pupil of the eye, it is the pattern being looked at. In the experiment, to be sure that the infant was truly interested and not looking at the picture by chance, the pictures were reversed every ten seconds; each time, the observer checked and recorded which pattern was directly over the pupils.

From these observations, Dr. Fantz demonstrated that infants show preferences even among abstract patterns and are especially attracted to sharp outlines and to light and dark contrasts. If the pattern is dark, newborns are apt to search for light areas; if it is light, they search for dark areas. Both eyes actually look in the direction of the pattern, and the baby shows attention not only by looking, but also by lifting the upper eyelid—by "brightening" the eye. If babies are sucking on a bottle while watching the pattern, they will cease to suck. Babies can also recognize and show interest in primary colors—red, blue, and yellow.

The newborn has an innate ability to select certain forms for longer examination. The tendency to look longer or more often at a particular picture or pattern indicates the capabilities of distinguishing among objects or patterns and expressing preferences. By patiently studying hundreds of babies, Dr. Fantz documented that infants look longer at—or prefer—patterns (circles and stripes) over plain surfaces. Further, they prefer complex patterns, with more elements, over simpler and less-detailed patterns. He later showed that infants also prefer curving rather than straight patterns.

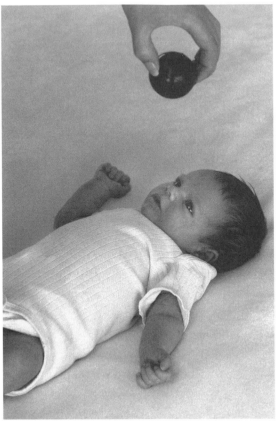

Infant looks directly at red ball.

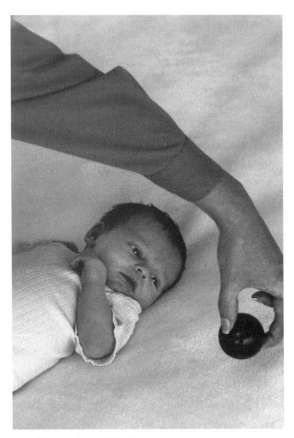

He follows the red ball.

The possibility that these selections might indicate an adaptive preference for human faces has long fascinated investigators. Do infants recognize the human face, or are they attracted simply to the contrast of features— eyes, hair, facial outline—with the background? This dispute has been investigated by asking whether, given a choice, an infant prefers a scrambled or an unscrambled face. Recent studies confirm that the infant is especially attracted to the normal face.

Through all these visual experiences the new baby is constantly learning. He takes in new images, encodes them in memory, begins to categorize them, and becomes familiar with them. Babies love to look at their parents' faces, which, in a short while, become of unwavering importance to them. At the same time, because their brains are geared for learning, for developing, and for making connections, babies are also interested in new objects and images.

Newborns are also especially attracted to

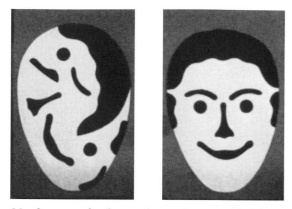

Newborns prefer the regular to the scrambled face.

movement. When a moving object catches their attention, they are apt to focus on it. They will follow it with their eyes and sometimes with their heads as well. If a red ball is moved slowly at a distance of ten inches from a baby's face, he will first follow it with his eyes and then turn his head horizontally and sometimes vertically. Initially, his attention will be intense, but after a few minutes he loses interest. The baby may turn away, and sometimes becomes drowsy, actually falls asleep, or tunes out an apparently uninteresting image. Some infants become locked in or hooked on what they are looking at and will stare at an object for periods of up to ten minutes. These distinct individual differences show up very early in life.

Because the ability to see and focus on visual objects occurs mainly during the quiet alert state, it can be overlooked by anyone not sensitive to a baby's cues. Also, because babies are born nearsighted, they cannot initially accommodate their vision to distances. Thus activity across a room will not catch their attention.

Newborn vision is best in a range of eight to ten inches from the face. This is not surprising, when we realize that this is about the same distance from which an infant views his mother's face during a feeding. If objects are moved too close or too far, they go out of focus and can be seen only as a haze or blur. To test an infant's ability to focus and follow, objects should be kept in that eight- to ten-inch range. Before you move the object, the baby should be looking directly at it and paying attention to it.

To build a three-dimensional world visually, the infant must see with both eyes. If the sight in one eye is impaired because the cornea (the clear covering of the eye) or the lens (behind the cornea) is cloudy, binocular, or stereo, vision will not develop. The neural connections in the visual system are made in these first three months and require the presence of good vision in both eyes. Therefore, any problem with vision should be picked up early and corrected. The baby's ability to see smaller and finer detail with more clarity and sharpness improves over the next three months and continues to improve over the next few years. However, newborns do see well enough to imitate and respond to rather intricate facial expressions and to be attracted to the details in their parents' faces. Even this early, babies are especially responsive to subtle changes of feelings in their mother's face.

Newborns tend to scan the outer contours of patterns rather than look at inner details. When they look at human faces, they usually scan the outline and then move to the eyes and mouth.

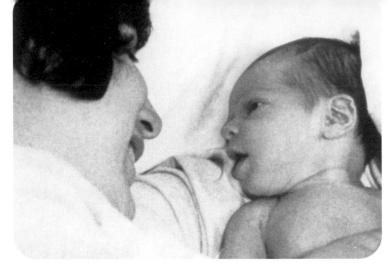

Video shots capture a newborn as she begins to follow the outline of her mother's face.

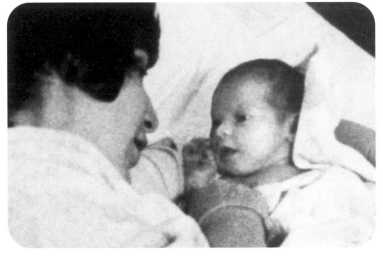

She now looks at her mother's mouth and lifts her hand.

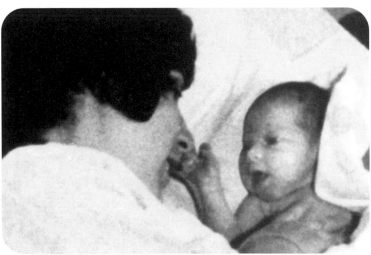

She reaches to touch what she sees.

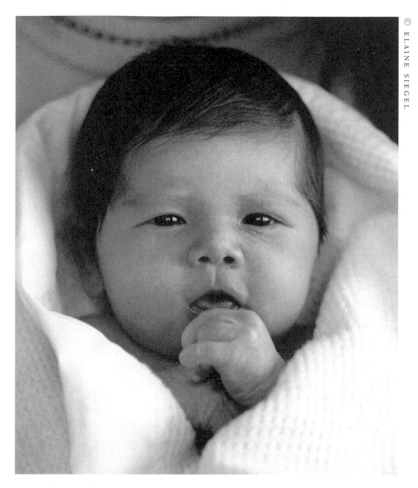

A newborn taking in her mother

Eyes are particularly engrossing to the infant. In the sequence shown here, a baby just a few hours old scans her mother's face and then reaches to touch what she is looking at (an unusual example of the coordination of touch and vision). To reach for the mouth requires the capacity to see the details of the mother's face.

In the quiet alert state, as the eyes become bright and wide open, the infant will often stop moving or sucking and become very still. These short periods of rapt visual attention, occurring shortly after birth and throughout this early period, draw the newborn into eye-to-eye contact, a vital element in human interaction. In this mutual gaze, the first dialogue begins; both parent and child seem magnetically drawn into communication.

Interesting visual objects can change an

infant's state of consciousness. A drowsy or crying baby can become quietly alert if something fascinating catches his eye. The state of quiet alertness can sometimes be increased or maintained by changing what a baby is able to see from his bassinet or crib.

Newborns are also capable of processing visual information, remembering what they have seen, and using that information. When shown a series of pictures on different parts of a screen, they soon began to anticipate another picture and look in the direction from which it might be coming before it appears. Another study demonstrated that if infants are shown the same picture for a long period of time, they tend to decrease their looking time, as if bored. When shown a new and different picture, they demonstrate renewed interest. This is called response to novelty, and may signify an early ability to remember a picture already seen. When babies are given a series of pairs of pictures of faces to look at, they show equal interest in two new pictures, but when a new picture is paired with a previously seen picture, they show much more interest in the new face. This is further evidence of the infant's ability to remember.

If a mother wears a mask on her face when her infant is eight days old, her infant will recognize the change and look at her frequently during feedings as if something is wrong or different. This same infant will take less milk, and when placed down to nap will be restless and will not fall asleep quickly. The baby will also sleep for a shorter period of time. This evidence suggest that newborns can recognize their

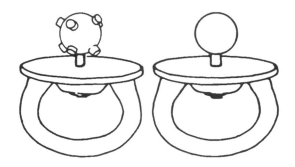

Pebbly and smooth pacifiers

mother and actually remember her face. Even a subtle change, such as adding dark-rimmed glasses, can make a baby appear quite puzzled.

Such feats of visual perception and memory by the baby indicate that the infant's visual talent is based not only on reflex eye movement, but on higher brain function as well. The baby is learning where to look, what to expect; he is taking in information about the sequence of events and making choices about what to look at. When alert, babies not only can see, but they look about spontaneously. They can even recognize depth and may respond with a defensive reaction to approaching objects.

One of the most remarkable feats of the infant is matching information coming in from two different senses. This ability to process and store abstract information about objects has been studied mainly in three-week-old infants. Either a smooth or pebbly pacifier was slipped into the babies' mouths without letting them see what it looked like. The babies were given a minute and a half to become familiar with the

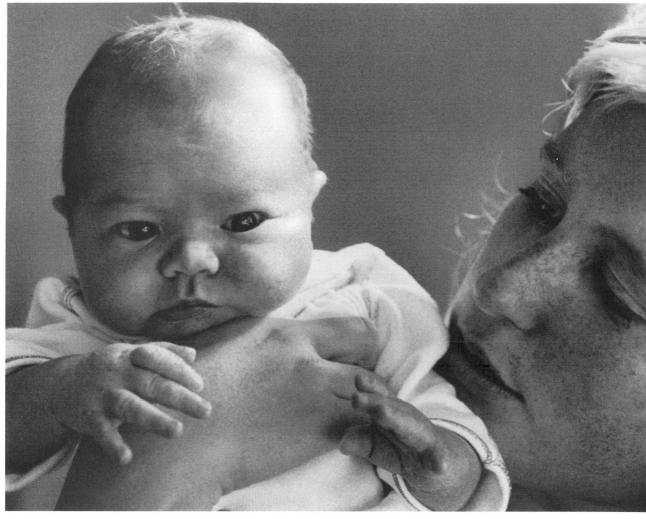

A mother learning about her two-hour-old baby as the baby begins to explore her surroundings

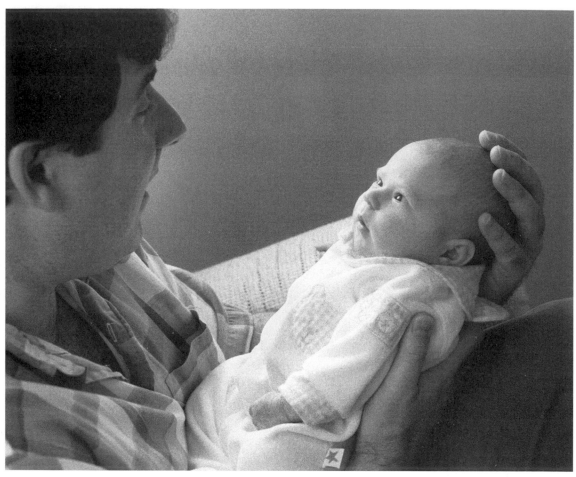

Three-day-old girl and her father in a mutual gaze

pacifier. The pacifiers were then slipped out of their mouths, again remaining out of sight. The babies were then briefly shown two pictures of pacifiers, one pebbly and one smooth. An observer looked through a peephole at the images in the pupils, as in Dr. Fantz's experiment, to see which picture the babies preferred. The majority of babies looked at the picture of the pacifier they had had in their mouth. This finding suggests that somewhere in their brains, the infants were able to match the sensations they received from mouthing the object with other sensations they received when looking at the object—an incredible achievement for the brain of a human infant.

The newborn's visual curiosity and ability to have eye-to-eye contact is, of course, very rewarding for parents and caretakers. Because

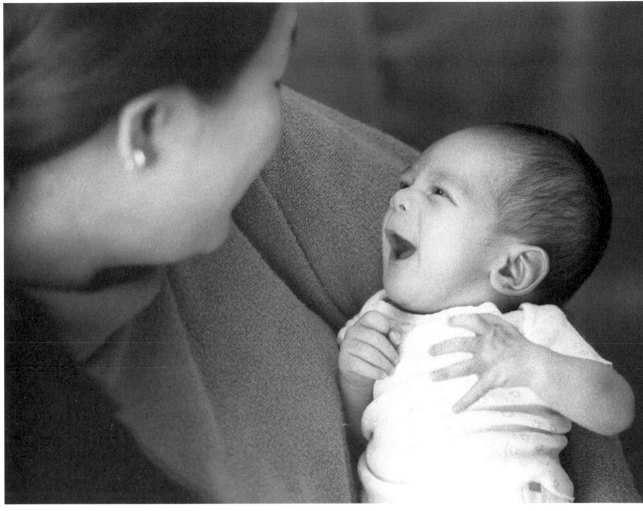

Week-old boy and his mother sharing a moment of joy

infants blink less than do adults, they have a wondrous, staring sort of gaze or look. Along with other infant facial features, such as a prominent forehead and chubby cheeks, these large, inquiring eyes are especially appealing. Just as babies seem born with a preference for human faces, adults may be programmed to enjoy and be drawn to small babies.

A baby's early visual ability and parents' insatiable desire to admire their baby draw them close and help them begin the long adventure of learning about one another.

NEWBORN 5 HEARING

Sound travels easily through the womb, and months before birth, babies' sense of hearing is already acute and well developed. On an ultrasound screen, fetuses have been observed to startle at loud sounds as early as the twenty-fifth or twenty-sixth week of pregnancy. Newborns can distinguish types of sounds (for example, a buzzer from a bell), loudness and pitch (frequency), different voices, and familiar and unfamiliar sounds. They can even determine the direction from which sound is coming.

Newborn babies prefer high-pitched voices, and mothers and fathers seem instinctively to use high-pitched voices when they first talk to their babies after delivery. Such baby talk seems to be a universal phenomenon. Patricia Kuhl, a neuroscientist at the University of Washington, has shown that mothers of several nationalities use a similar kind of "parentese," or exaggerated speech, in talking to their newborns.

Infants respond to sounds from inanimate sources as well. When a small bell is rung, they will turn their eyes and then their head in the direction of the sound. Orienting to sound is something humans do without thinking. Our heads are like antennae moving automatically into position for the best reception. Newborns start to do this from the first moments after birth; they look to the right when the sound is coming from the right and to the left when the

sound is coming from the left. The nerves connecting vision and hearing are already developed in the newborn.

This ability to look toward the source of the sound may be part of the infant's attempt to get better reception, or perhaps this eye-and-ear response is one of the many built-in connections between two or more senses, an adaptive response that ensures experiencing the environment as fully as possible.

Babies not only can make associations between sound and other senses, but also can be taught to respond in different ways to the same sound and, if permitted, will exert some control in choosing sounds they want to hear. For instance, one-day-old infants learned to turn their head to the right at the sound of a bell; they also learned not to turn their head to the right at the sound of a buzzer. This complex response was achieved by rewarding the babies with sugar water only when they responded to the bell. They were then taught the reverse, which they learned very quickly; that is, they turned their head to the right only for the buzzer, not for the bell, after having been rewarded with sugar water only when the buzzer sounded. The ability to make associations from different sensory input at such an early age may represent a fundamental process of human learning.

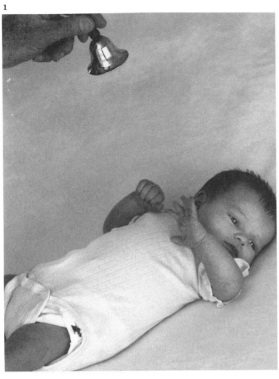

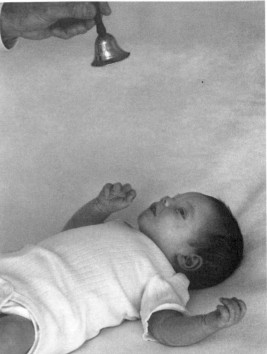

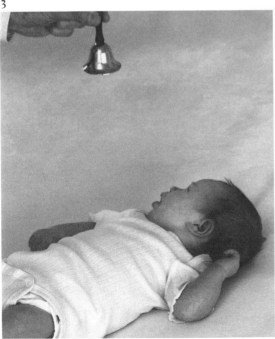

1 *Infant begins to hear a bell.*

2 *He turns in the direction of the sound.*

3 *He follows the sound.*

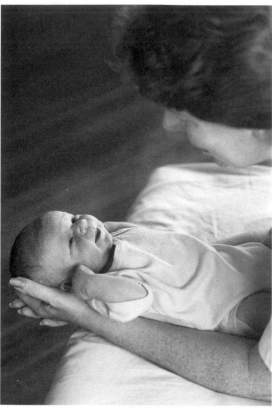

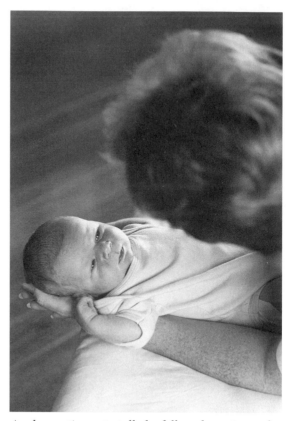

Mother engages her son with her voice and face.

As she continues to talk, he follows her voice and face.

Researchers have also asked whether infants can coordinate the hand and the ear in the same way in which they coordinate the hand and the eye. Can they reach for an object using the sense of sound, instead of relying only on sight as a guide to the object's location? Researchers surmised that because infants are generally passive recipients of sound and cannot turn away from sounds in the environment as one would turn away from sights (or close the eyes), they may not develop or use the sensory connection between hearing and touch. Since

babies exert no active control over what they hear, they might lose interest, become habituated, or lose the motivation or the need to use this skill.

T. G. R. Bower at the University of Edinburgh designed a device that would give infants control over the sounds they heard. He used earphones with ultrasonic receivers that transmitted different audible sounds to the infant depending on the position of the baby's head in relationship to different objects. One study with a blind infant illustrated that the infant could

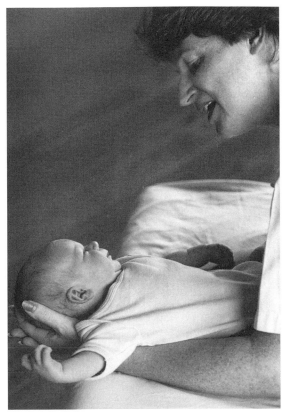

She moves to the other side, still talking, and he follows her voice and face.

detect an object in front of him when the sonic device indicated that the object was present. The infant raised his hands as if he had seen the object. These different perceptual skills are present at birth and continue to evolve and develop with time. The newborn has a variety of ways to perceive her world and learns to use them according to the situation.

Infants are most responsive to human voices. Parents can have fun with their baby when she is in a quiet alert state by talking a short distance from her ear in a soft, high-pitched voice. At first the baby's eyes may turn in the direction of her parent's voice, and almost simultaneously, her head will turn, her face brighten, and her eyes open a bit wider. Even more appealing to the infant is being talked to while exchanging mutual looks.

Although newborns respond to inanimate sounds, such as a bell, for a short time, they recognize and prefer human speech. They also seem to have a built-in preference for a live voice speaking to them with feeling over a voice on the radio, for example. The desire for human verbal responses dovetails with the baby's emotional need to be loved and cuddled. However, the baby's delight in hearing a real-life voice talking to her fades when the same voice, even if it is her mother's voice, reads a text backward, without any emotional tone or meaning. When sounds become mechanical, the baby loses interest.

Discovering these preferences has required considerable ingenuity on the part of investigators. Dr. Anthony DeCasper, an early leader in this research, recognized that since infants have superb innate control of their mouths and lips, they might be able to indicate a preference by changing their sucking rate or tempo. He contrived the following experiment. Working with one- to two-day-old infants in the alert state, Dr. DeCasper placed a nipple in the mouth of each baby and fitted the baby with a pair of padded earphones. The nipple was attached to a device that triggered different recordings. For example, when the infant sucked at a high rate, she would hear a recording of a woman's voice, and

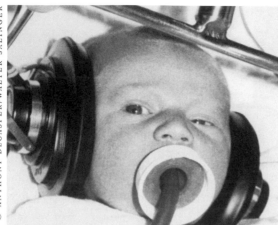

DeCasper placed padded earphones on this day-old girl and arranged for her to control what she heard by changing her sucking rate.

when she sucked at a low rate, she would hear a man's recorded voice. Almost all infants quickly learned that their sucking rate determined what they heard. Eleven of twelve babies tested in this manner sucked at the high rate to hear the woman's voice. To be sure that this was not just related to preferring to suck at a high rate, the woman's high-pitched voice was alternated, so that for some of the babies it was heard when they sucked at a low rate. The results showed a similar preference. Here were one- and two-day-old babies controlling their environment just as adults control their environment when they turn on Mozart instead of rock music.

Using similar techniques, Dr. DeCasper found that infants prefer their own mother's voice over other women's voices. Although the same preference for their own father's voice was not seen at first, later investigators found that, in the week after birth, 80 percent of babies come to prefer their father's voice to that of another male. Their preference for their mother's voice may be the enduring result of continually hearing their mother's voice during fetal life, or it might possibly be due to the fact that at normal conversational levels, male voices are less easily distinguishable through the uterine wall because of their lower pitch. Just as exposure to loud noise over a period of time in pregnancy can be a danger to the fetus, high noise levels have been shown to cause hearing loss in newborns.

As we said earlier, most sound penetrates into the womb. A French obstetrician investigated prenatal hearing by placing a very small microphone into the uterus while mothers were in labor (after the membranes had broken) and recording the intensity of the sound that reached the infant. He also observed a variety of different responses (heart rate and movement, for example) that babies made to different types of sounds. Most sounds penetrated the uterine and abdominal walls. In one such experiment, the physician could hear not only the unmistakable sounds and levels of voices in the room and the mother's internal body sounds, but also Beethoven's Ninth Symphony, which was being played in the delivery suite!

Many people have wondered if this capacity to pick up and respond to sound during fetal life might influence musical preferences or ability, as well as account for the infant's response to and familiarity with her mother's voice. Many great composers had parents who were musicians. Of course, the experience of early childhood could just as well be the key factor, not to mention lessons, hard work, and talent.

We spoke to a mother and father who were rehearsing for roles in two different operas while the mother was pregnant. At the birth, the father welcomed his daughter into the world singing an aria. Within the first hour, according to her parents, she made little sounds, "uh, uh," apparently making an effort to mimic or respond to the sounds she was hearing. Later, at home, her parents noticed these same efforts— "ah, ah, uh, uh"—and within a few weeks they could detect a difference in tone in these sounds. Their little girl would easily quiet after crying when she heard music either from records or from her parents' singing. Many parents have reported similar experiences, though it will always be difficult to disentangle genetic tendencies, prenatal experience, and early nurture of talent.

What is the influence of intrauterine experiences in relation to later hearing and sound production? To learn whether babies have any memory of what they heard in utero, Dr. DeCasper and his colleagues did another series of intriguing studies. They initially tape-recorded each of sixteen mothers while the women read both *The Cat in the Hat* and a poem called "The King, the Mice and the Cheese." During the last six and a half weeks of their pregnancy, each mother in the study was asked to read aloud only one of these children's stories to her fetus, which she did twice a day. Thus each fetus had a total of about five hours of listening time to the same story read over and over until birth. At three days of age, padded earphones were placed on the babies' ears and the recordings of both of these stories were played to them. The babies heard one story if they sucked rapidly and the other story if they sucked slowly. Amazingly, fifteen of sixteen sucked at the right rate to receive the story they had heard their mothers read over and over again when they were fetuses—not too different from the requests of a toddler to hear again and again a favorite story!

When medical students are first introduced to newborn babies, they are always surprised at the alacrity of the responses the babies give their mother in comparison with their manner of responding to a stranger. The babies become quiet at the sound of their mother's voice and almost immediately begin to turn their head. It has been shown that infants are already coordinating sight, sound, and the memory of their mother's voice within the first two weeks after birth. Mothers in one study were fascinated to learn that their infants showed much confusion and distress when hearing their mother's voice apparently coming from another woman's face or saw their mother's face while they heard another woman's voice. The infants showed comfort only when the situation was corrected.

The infant's reaction to certain familiar sounds after birth depends on the stage of fetal life during which that sound was heard. When fetuses under six months' gestation are

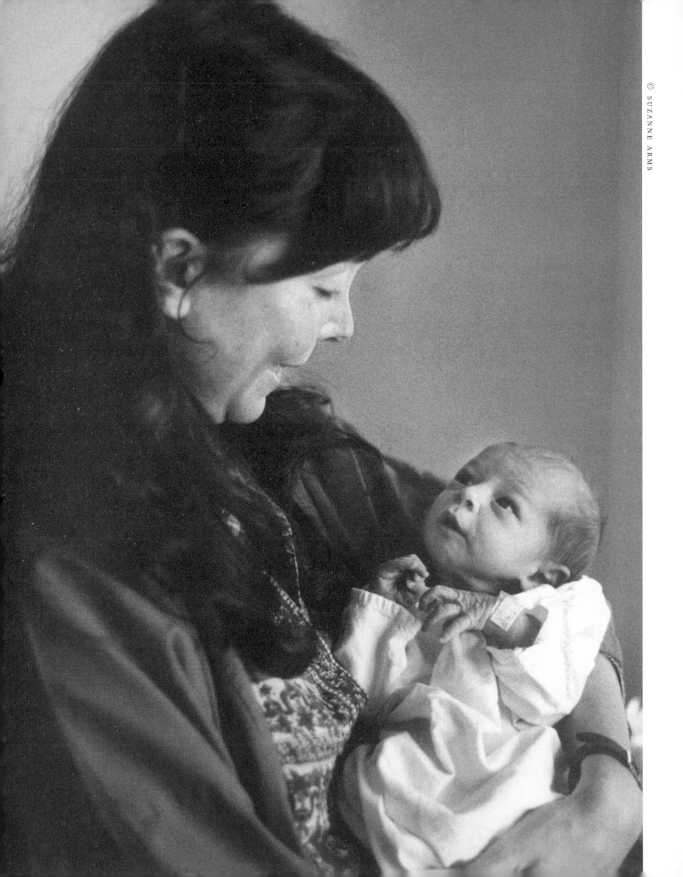

repeatedly subjected to the loud noises of an airplane taking off, they adapt in such a way that in the first days after birth they will sleep right through those sounds. But when fetuses hear the same loud noises continually at a point later than seven months in the womb, after birth they react with distress to those noises. In contrast, as just discussed, a mother's frequent reading of a pleasant story late in pregnancy may result in her newborn's desire to hear the same story read over and over again.

The infant's brain is capable of taking in a multitude of vocalizations and eventually categorizing and making meaning out of them. Babies can distinguish minute differences in spoken sounds, in pitch, and in rhythms. They also prefer approving speech (soft and melodious) to angry (sharp, strong, abrupt) vocalizations. These developing capacities in the infants correspond to parents' typical ways of speaking to them—the parentese studied in depth by Patricia Kuhl, mentioned earlier. This way of talking highlights, magnifies, and prolongs vowel sounds and uses a higher pitch, which babies prefer. Giving more attention to vowel and other particular sounds enables infants to develop more familiarity with the sounds in their native language and helps them as they learn to understand that language.

In every language, certain basic themes must be learned in order to create words. For the first few months all babies can distinguish and respond to the various sounds of any language. By six months, infants appear to analyze and categorize sounds particular to their native language, and after a while, they do not react to minor differences in the common vowel sounds to which they have become accustomed, but will show a distinct reaction to a nonfamiliar, or foreign, language sound. This complex learning takes place whether the language is English, with nine vowels; Russian, with five; Swedish, with sixteen; or Japanese, with its own distinct sounds of vowels and consonants. The inherent motivation for learning and responding on the part of the infant and the natural effort to teach on the part of parents come together in a powerful way to develop communication.

◀ *An early conversation*

TOUCH, TASTE, AND SMELL

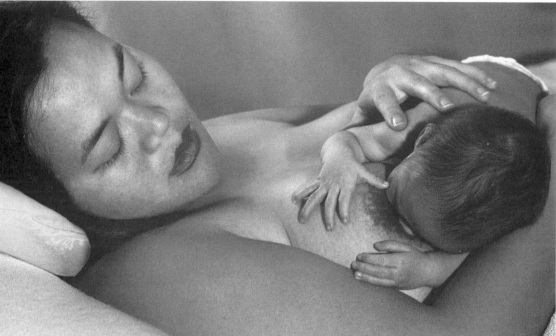

Soon after birth, an infant enjoys touch, taste, and smell.

The sense of touch is activated well before birth, since babies are surrounded and caressed by warm fluid and tissues from the beginning of fetal life. After birth, they continue to like closeness, warmth, and tactile comforting. Babies generally like to be cuddled and will often nestle and mold to your body. Parents all over the world naturally lift, hold, stroke, rock, and walk with their infant, using a great variety of touch-

ing motions to soothe him. Both parent and infant seem prepared to enjoy this experience.

Newborns respond to other aspects of touch as well: variations in temperature, texture, moisture, pressure, pain. Our lips and hands have the largest number of touch receptors, which may account for why newborns enjoy sucking their fingers. As we saw in Chapter 1, hands are frequently in close contact with the face from

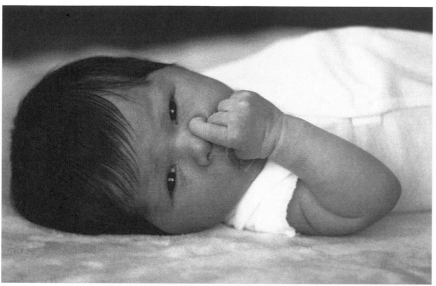

Self-soothing using two different techniques

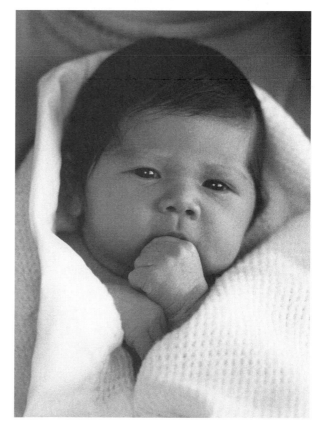

the fourteenth to the thirty-sixth week of fetal life. Fetuses suck their thumbs as early as twenty-four weeks. The sense of touch is a major component of how babies comfort themselves, explore their world, and initiate contact.

The skin is the largest sense organ in the body, and touch has many more benefits than previously recognized. Observations over many decades have shown that infants who are fed, but not held, touched, or interacted with, fail to thrive and their physical and mental development is severely slowed. Appropriate touch and massage apparently activate a variety of physiological as well as emotional responses that can soothe, relax, and enhance growth and comfort in infants. Touch has been demonstrated to increase production of growth hormones and aid the immune system. Mothers who practice daily infant massage describe much less distress and better sleep patterns in their infants. Although many different factors lead to colic in an infant, massage appears to reduce the symptoms.

Since the person who gives the massage receives as many benefits as the person experiencing it, it is no wonder that mothers and babies find mutual pleasure and closeness in this activity. Not only does massage help babies to sleep, but parents may find their own sleep improved as well, an unexpected and welcome benefit during a period that is often marked by sleep deprivation.

The influence of massage has been demonstrated even more dramatically in premature infants. Gentle and firm massage for fifteen minutes just three times a day results in nearly 50 percent more weight gain and better performance on tests of motor control and orientation to people. The improved growth appears to be the result of increased gastrointestinal hormones, which in turn increase the absorbing surfaces of the intestines for the nutrients from milk. Trained observers found that infants who received massage were more alert and active than were control infants who received the same daily caloric intake but no massage. In addition, the massaged premature infants went home from the hospital six days earlier.

There are many ways for parents to enjoy touch with their infant besides massage, such as holding, soothing, and carrying. Infant-carrying devices, such as slings or front carriers, help parents learn about their baby's responses, needs, and signals as well as give a sense of security to the baby. Infants whose needs are met appropriately and consistently in early life more frequently form a secure attachment to their parents and develop a basic trust in their world.

Taste is also highly developed in infants at birth. Observations of what newborns choose to suck have shown that infants are able to make fine discriminations and are responsive even to small chemical alterations in the foods placed on their tongues. Infants show pleasure as sweetness is increased and show displeasure when given slightly salty, acidic, or bitter liquids. Some of these preferences are developed in the womb; others are evident at birth; and still others develop over time.

Taste cells start to appear at seven to eight

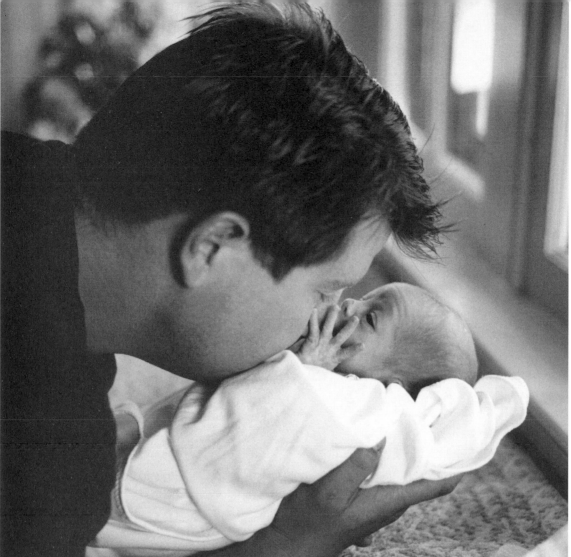

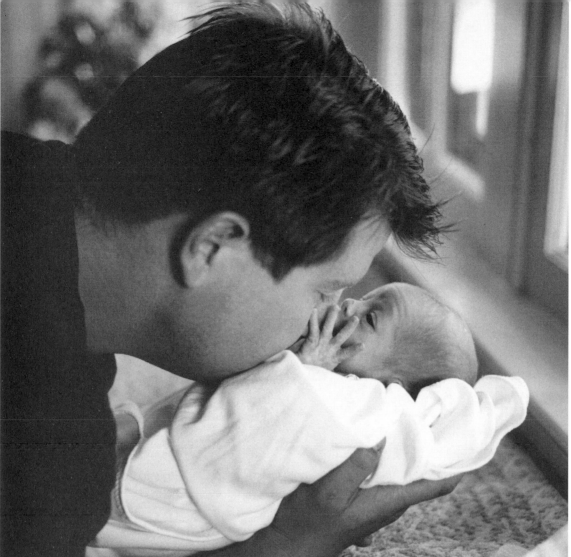

Many senses are involved in this single tender encounter.

weeks' gestation and begin to mature by four-teen weeks. They are stimulated by the various spices and chemicals circulating in the amniot-ic fluid that is swallowed frequently by the fetus during intrauterine life. At birth, some babies' bodies have been found to hold the odor of a particularly spicy food that the mother was eat-ing right before delivery. In this way, the fetus may receive an early introduction to the foods of its family and later, when starting to eat fin-ger foods, the baby may be willing to try new foods from the cuisine of the household. Simple tests with preterm infants show their preference for a very sweet taste. Within hours after birth, full-term newborns show their sophisticated preference for very sweet, sugary

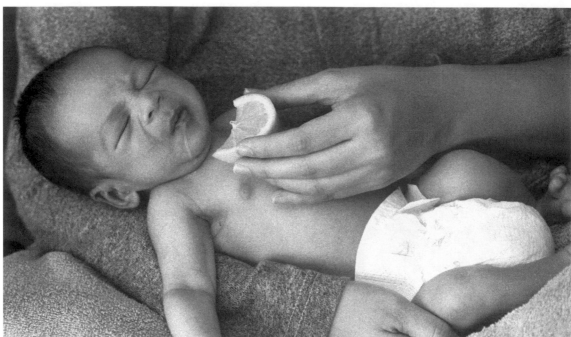

A pronounced reaction

tastes over mildly sweet sugars. When tasting the sweeter sugars, their faces relax and they continue sucking enthusiastically.

Newborns respond with expressions of rejection, such as grimacing or pursing their lips, for sour tastes, such as lemon, as well as for strong bitter tastes. At this early period they seem to be indifferent to the other basic tastes: mildly bitter, salty, or savory. Interest in a salty taste appears at about four months of age, and over the next twenty-four months more subtle differences in taste emerge. When first exposed to garlic through his mother's breast milk, the baby increases his milk intake, whereas a similar exposure to alcohol through breast milk causes the baby to decrease his milk intake. The four basic tastes—sweet, sour, bitter, and salty—detected by our tongue are hardwired in our brains, probably an adaptive benefit, since mother's milk is sweet, poisons are often bitter, and salt constitutes a major part of our bodies' fluids.

Flavor is the result of a summation from taste receptors around the tongue and the back of the throat and smell receptors (olfactory) in the back upper portion of the nose and the throat. The sense of smell plays a major role in the pleasurable sensations we derive from tastes. We have all experienced a diminished sense of taste during a severe head cold.

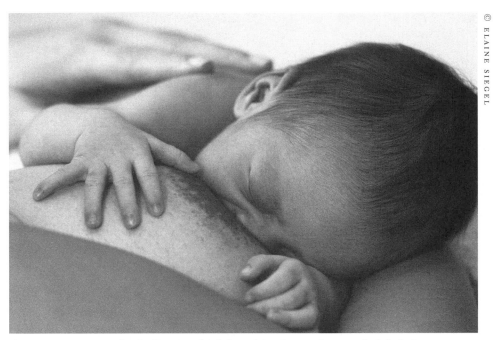

A common position for feeding in which breathing is not obstructed. A baby's nose adapts for this position.

Babies can distinguish and recognize different smells. After initially responding to new smells, they quickly adapt and stop responding once the smell becomes familiar. When a novel smell is presented, they show their interest by moving their heads; their activity level and heart rate change. By one to two days of life, breast-fed babies will recognize the smell of their own mother's breast pad and the odors from her neck and underarms compared with similar odors from another woman. To study this, researchers used small gauze pads—the type that women who are breast-feeding use to absorb leaking milk. On one side of the infant's face they placed a pad worn by the mother; on the other side they placed a clean pad or a pad worn by another mother. By one to two days of age, babies turned far more often to their mother's breast pad than to a clean breast pad or the breast pad of another mother. To be sure that the turning was not accidental, the location of the pads was changed frequently. The babies continued to turn toward their mother's pad. This preference became even more pronounced as the baby became older. Interestingly, though, when the mother's breast milk was placed on an unworn pad, the infants showed no preference. Apparently, the babies respond to the special smell of the mother herself, not necessarily to the smell of the milk.

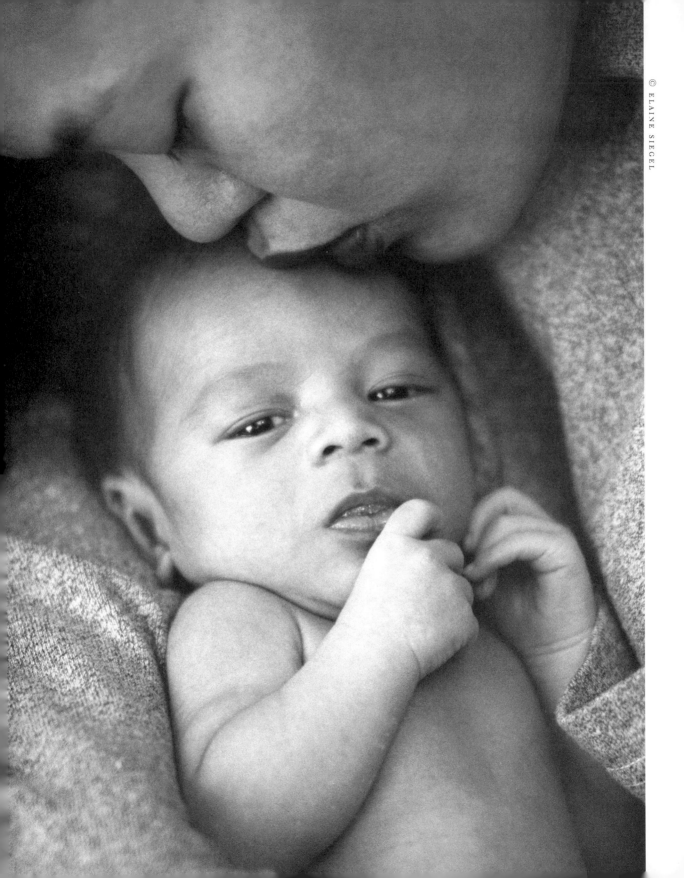

Bottle-fed infants show less ability to discriminate their mother's odors from those of other nonlactating women. Does the increased time the breast-feeding baby is skin to skin with his mother explain this ability to recognize her odors? Both breast- and bottle-fed infants appear to be drawn by the odors of the breast. Perhaps this preference may have had an adaptive advantage when breast milk was the only food available.

The baby's sensory capacities keep growing from the moment of birth. They can be nurtured or overloaded. When infants are pushed too much, on the one hand, or deprived of various sensory stimuli, on the other, their development may be affected. No one knows whether certain senses need to be enhanced or left alone. Clearly, however, infants take delight and interest in a variety of experiences. There is no right or perfect way to interact with them. By being attuned to their own infant, mothers and fathers soon learn what interests and amuses him and are able to discover enjoyable ways to interact.

◀ *An unfolding experience of closeness*

MOTIONS AND RHYTHMS 7

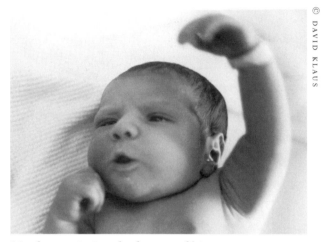

Newborn enjoying the free use of his arms.

At birth, the movements of a newborn appear jerky and random. These seemingly purposeless movements contain identifiable rhythms and patterns and lay a foundation for more deliberate action. Using the technique of time-lapse photography, taking one picture every second, much has been learned about infant motion. For instance, when awake and not crying, a baby's movement follows a very specific pattern. For about one and a quarter minutes, there is no movement at all; then there is a burst of movement, followed by a quiet period. This cycle of activity and stillness occurs continuously every one to two minutes when a newborn is in the active alert state of consciousness.

In contrast, reflexive startles or jerks sometimes occur in response to an external stimulus. The intrinsic rhythm to an infant's spontaneous arm and leg movements suggests that there may be a clock in each infant's brain that directs this system. The same type of spontaneous fluctuations in movement begin in the fetus as early as twenty weeks.

The amount of movement varies for each baby, with some infants moving much more or less than others; therefore, the range of total movement among normal newborns is large. While it is difficult to observe any pattern of activity without special films, this rhythmic motion probably accounts for a large amount of the activity in the early months of life.

With light pressure on an infant's palms, her mouth opens (the Babkin reflex).

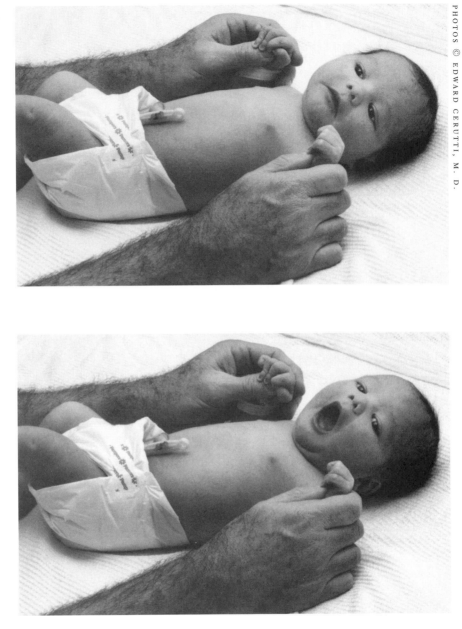

Some of these movements appear to be a reaching out and drawing in of arms and legs, as though they might be an invitation from the baby for the adult to play and respond.

Not only do individual babies show differences in their activity levels, responses, and personalities, but cultural practices and racial background also affect how much a baby moves. For example, when babies are swaddled, they become quiet and move little. Physical differences appear to be present at birth. Observations of black, white, and Asian newborns show that Asian infants tend to have less muscle strength at birth than do other infants. In comparison, black infants in general have the most muscle strength of the three groups. Muscle strength of white infants falls somewhere in between. As infants in all three groups grow, however, they develop a similar range of abilities.

For some time it has been recognized that newborns move their bodies in synchrony to adult speech. Almost imperceptibly, a newborn baby's body moves in rhythm with her mother's voice, performing a kind of dance as her mother talks. The movements of this dance are subtle. They might consist of the slight motion of an eyebrow lifting, a foot extending, or an arm raising. Each syllable may elicit a new movement. The infant's moving body parts are coordinated with the elements of speech, even including the pauses or changes in the sound patterns. Such synchronous movements can be detected only by filming using special techniques. Newborns are somehow programmed to respond to human speech; tapping noises and disconnected vowel sounds do not elicit corresponding movements.

Adults in all societies respond nonverbally as well as verbally to one another's speech. Listeners to any conversation move their bodies in rhythm with the speaker. We do not consciously recognize these nonverbal movements, but we perceive, or receive, them at an unconscious or subliminal level, and they may engage us to continue the communication. The movements are a signal from the listener that he or she is aware of what we are saying. When a mother believes that her baby is responding to her, the two are actually in tune with one another. A baby's body is prepared for a conversation long before she can say any words.

Many other responses in a newborn are, in large part, automatic and are termed *reflexes*. For instance, when you press your thumb into an infant's palm, the baby's mouth opens; this is known as the Babkin reflex. If you stroke an infant's cheek, she will turn in that direction and open her mouth. An infant comes into the world ready to eat, and this rooting reflex makes it easier to begin the feeding.

The grasping reflex is very strong. Newborns can even hold their own weight under certain circumstances and with help will pull to a sitting position. Some scientists think that this reflex represents an evolutionary adaptation because it would have allowed the infant to hold onto the mother's hair during prolonged hikes or while escaping from danger. A baby's toes attempt to grasp in a similar fashion. The

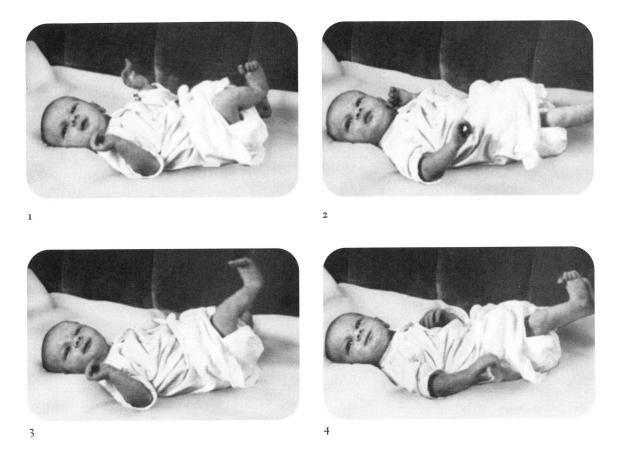

Video shots of an infant girl listening to a voice saying "pre-tty ba-by." Her body moves in rhythm to speech.

1   "Pre": The baby's arms and feet pull back on the first syllable.

2   "Tty": Her feet extend and her right arm swings down on the second syllable.

3   "Ba": The baby's legs lift up and her arms pull back on the third syllable.

4   "By": With the last syllable, her mouth closes, her feet extend once more, a big toe wiggles, and both arms lower.

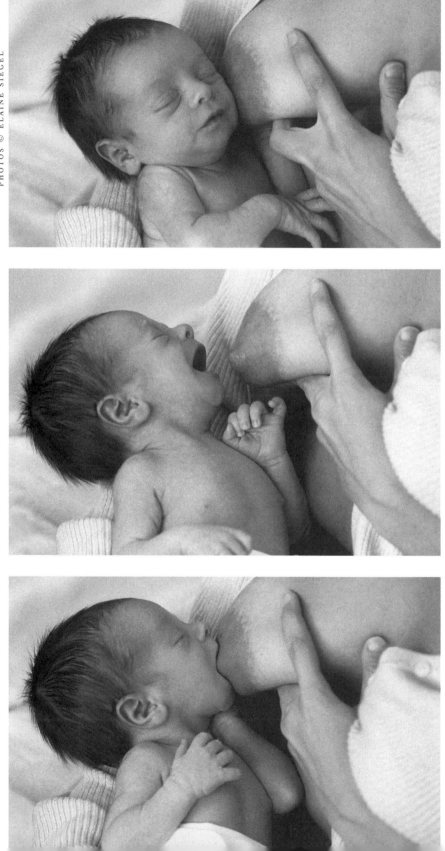

Mother initiates the rooting reflex in her infant boy.

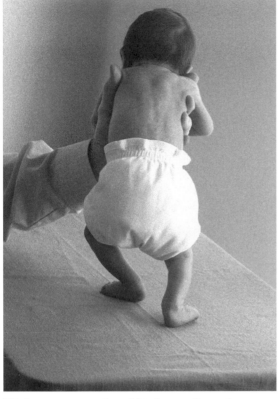

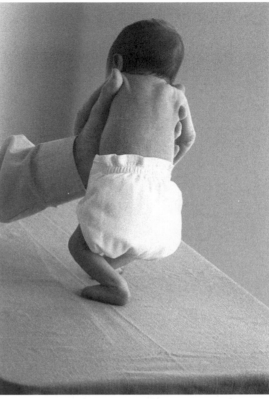

With support, a 2 day old infant walks, using one foot and then the other. Note that he is moving closer to far end of table, step by step.

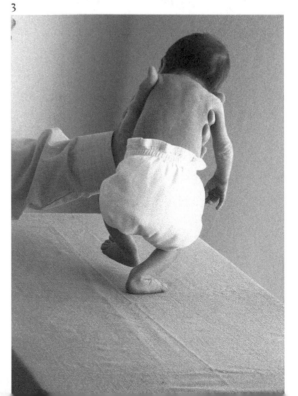

well-known Moro reflex is seen when the infant is put down suddenly or startled; her arms and legs shoot out abruptly and then inward slightly. Another automatic motion occurs when infants are held upright with their feet touching the top of a table; they make stepping movements, as though they were about to walk.

Infants share other automatic reflexes with adults. Their heart responds to emotional changes, such as fear, with an increased heart rate. They sneeze if their nose is tickled with a

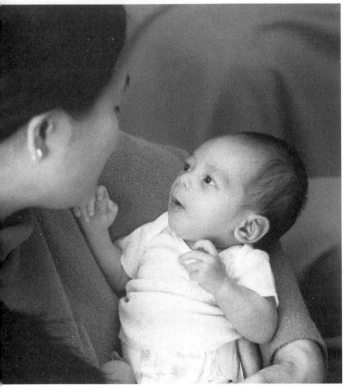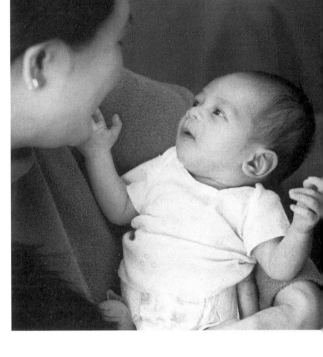

Reaching for his mother's face

feather, cough and gag when food goes down the wrong way, and often have a large bowel movement after a big meal. They also have formidable yawns.

The random, reflex arm and leg movements of a baby in the active alert state have made many experts believe that newborns are too immature to have the capacity to reach for objects. This theory was invalidated when two French pediatricians demonstrated that some newborns could reach. When in the quiet alert state, in a supported position, and being communicated with, some babies will reach.

Normal newborns at birth apparently have the underlying potential to reach. However, their very strong neck muscles are linked to their arms, so that a slight movement of the neck moves their arms as well. This connection protects the baby's head from suddenly dropping forward or backward, but it also prevents the baby from deliberately reaching unless the neck muscles are very relaxed or the head is being held and kept from moving.

When we heard of the work of these pediatricians, we searched the films we had taken of parents and newborns interacting and realized

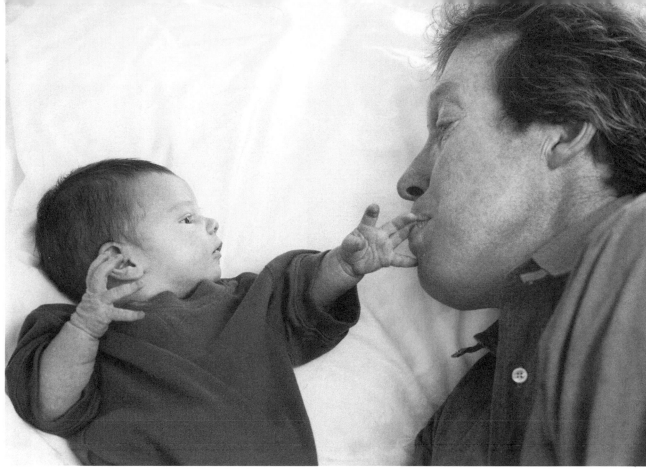

Infant reaching for his grandfather's face

that we had unknowingly filmed this reaching ability in two of the infants we had studied.

Running the films over and over in slow motion, we began to see signs of reaching. Twice we could see the baby's hand reach for the father's finger. Our belief that a newborn could not reach had kept us from seeing this before. This ability to reach is present until three to four weeks of age, then disappears until three and a half to four months, when it reappears permanently.

The photos on these pages catch such instances of reaching. Opportunities to observe this phenomenon sometimes arise; they require the right circumstances and an educated eye. Even the original French studies found reaching in only half of the normal babies tested. Although evidence of this ability is exciting, parents should know that trying to encourage reaching will not improve a baby's talents or abilities. (See also the pictures on page 34.)

We believe that the parents' own feelings and sensitivities to their infant's needs and pace form the ideal environment for the unfolding of the infant's natural development. We mention the ability to reach only to suggest that once in a

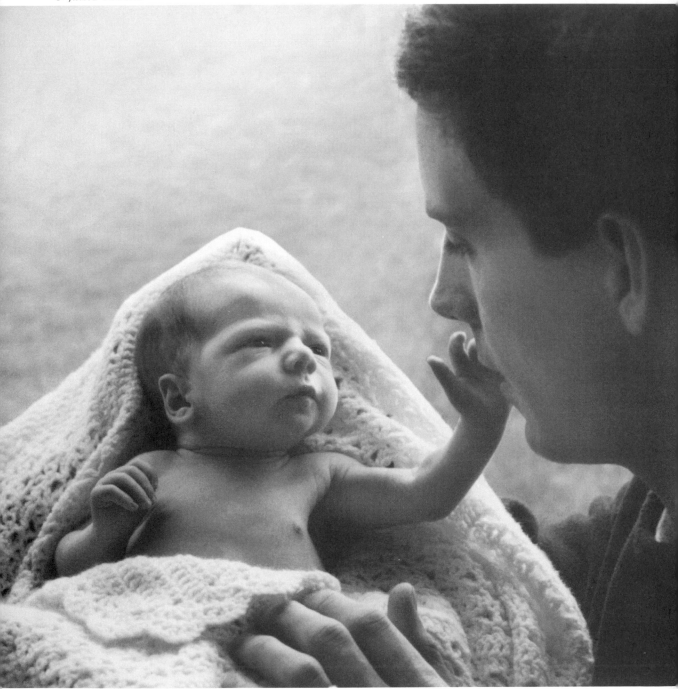

while, when playing a finger game with a baby, the baby may actually be reaching for the parent's finger rather than the reverse.

As parents watch their own baby's fascinating array of motions, patient attention will help sort them out. One set of wiggles could be the result of the automatic rhythm we mentioned, setting the newborn off every minute and a half. Certain repeated motions could be the result of automatic reflexes. More rhythmic patterns might indicate that the baby is moving in tune to words. On rare occasions, motion could reflect an attempt to reach out. Or, the baby may simply be moving an arm or leg because her position is uncomfortable. When the baby is asleep, as mentioned earlier, movement can mean that she is dreaming. Exploring these various motions and their meanings is another way of getting to know a newborn.

◀ *Newborn reaching to explore his father's face*

EXPRESSIONS *&* AND EMOTIONS

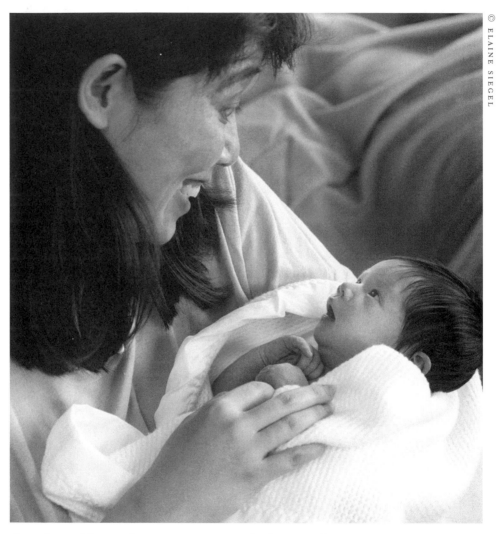

A mother and her newborn cannot get enough of one another.

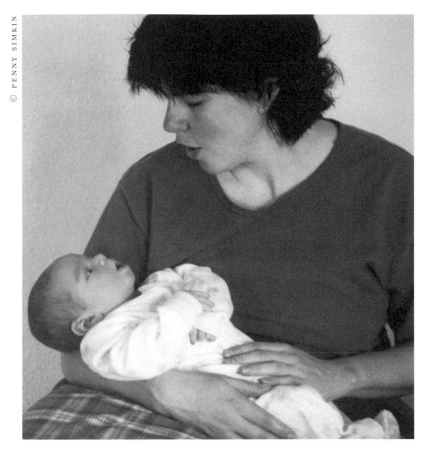

Infant girl imitating her mother

Babies' faces have a special fascination for most adults. The broad forehead, shiny eyes, tiny nose, and plump, soft cheeks are like a magnetic force that attracts men and women as well as children. Not surprisingly, tape recordings of mothers' reactions when alone for the first time with their infant reveal that nearly 80 percent of what they say relates to the face of the baby, especially the eyes.

Just as parents are interested in their baby's face, the baby, in turn, arrives in the world with a special fascination for faces. As we saw in Chapter 4, when newborns are shown comparisons of a human face and a scrambled face, they prefer the human face. When quiet and alert, babies will often gaze at their parents' faces with special interest or pleasure and are capable not only of responding to what they see, but also of imitating certain expressions.

Try this yourself. With the baby in a quiet alert state, about eight to ten inches away from you and looking directly at your face, slowly

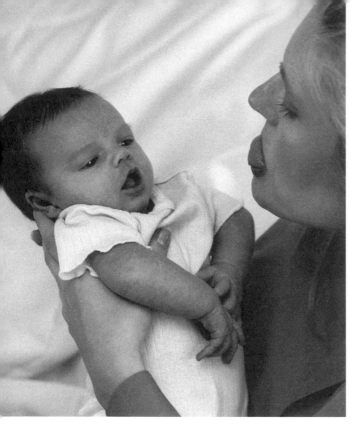

1 *Infant watching his mother*

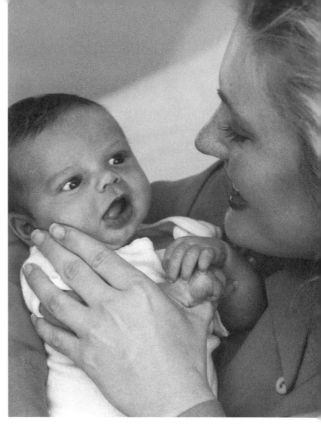

2 *Imitating his mother*

3 *Discovering his own tongue*

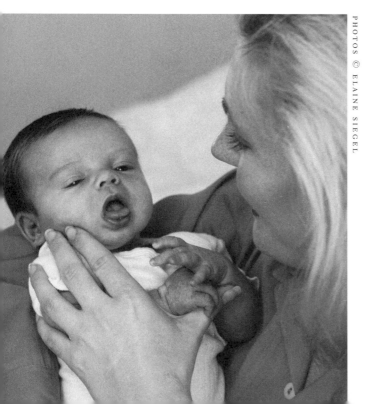

protrude your tongue as far as you can. Repeat the tongue protrusion slowly every twenty seconds, six to eight times; then stop. The baby, if he continues to look at your face, may begin to move his own tongue in his mouth. He may first move it against one inside cheek; then, after sixty or ninety seconds, his tongue will slowly appear at his lips, and, finally, may be pushed far out of the mouth. This will work only if you protrude your tongue while the baby's attention is on your face. A word of caution: babies have minds of their own and may not choose to play this game.

Some years ago, during a teaching visit to China, we observed an unusual example of this ability to imitate. While we were demonstrating a newborn's various talents, I asked a revered older professor to play the tongue-protrusion game with an eight-hour-old baby girl. As the professor slowly stuck out her tongue, then waited the appropriate time, the baby began to protrude her tongue. All twelve doctors and nurses present were delighted. Then I showed the baby around the circle one by one so the staff could view the infant face to face, and I asked the doctors and nurses not to stick out their tongues. When the baby again came face-to-face with the first professor, the baby immediately protruded her tongue, even though the professor made no facial expression or movements. Everyone gasped! We decided to try it again, after a pause. We went away from the baby to examine other infants, and then came back to the first baby. She stuck out her tongue only for the professor who had begun the game, and without any prompting! The memory trace of this professor appeared indelibly etched in the mind of that little newborn girl.

How do babies accomplish such a remarkable feat? They must somehow sense that they have a tongue as the other person does, as well as where it is located and how to control it. The act of imitation is a complex affair. It is wonderful to realize that a newborn infant—never having looked in a mirror, never having played the toddler game of finding his own or his parent's nose—somehow recognizes that what he is seeing in another's face relates to a part of his own body!

This game can affect the behavior of both parent and baby in strange ways. A mother described how, first, her baby yawned, inspiring her to yawn, then the baby yawned again, and so on, until they both fell asleep.

The facial expressions of newborns are strikingly similar across all cultures. It seems that when expressing the common emotions of fear, sadness, joy, disgust, and anger, the human face speaks a universal language. From the newborn period on, photographs of babies show that infants are capable of producing almost all the adult facial expressions of specific emotions.

Early studies of babies' imitation of emotions were done by Tiffany Field and her colleagues. An adult modeled a series of three facial expressions (sadness, happiness, and surprise) to a group of newborn infants. An observer standing behind the adult model was not able to view the

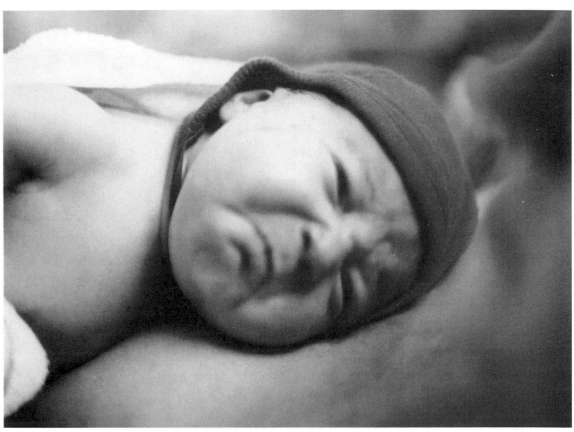

One hour old, this baby shows a sad expression.

model's face and therefore did not know which expressions were being demonstrated. As he watched, the observer noted on paper what facial expressions he thought the baby was imitating. The notes and the model's expressions matched remarkably often. (Both the infant's and the adult model's faces were videotaped to provide a later check on the observer's notations.)

Newborns focus their eyes on the eyes and mouth of the adult as they watch the adult's expressions. Infants will then change their own eyes and mouths according to what they see. Notice the widening of the eyes and the mouth when they imitate the expression of surprise, while they pull in the brows and protrude the mouth in imitation of the sad expression. It is not known when newborns experience inner

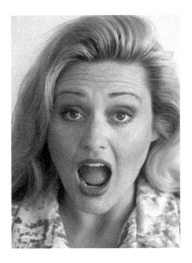

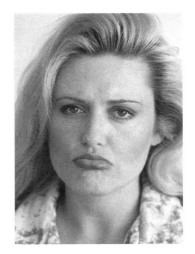

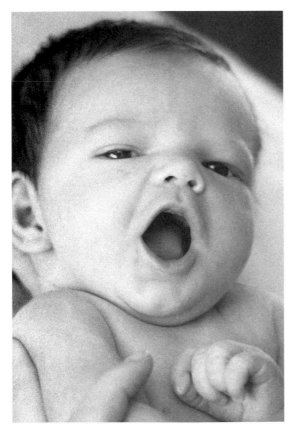

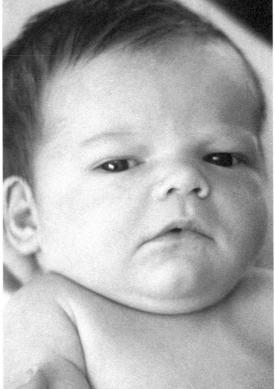

Infant imitating his mother

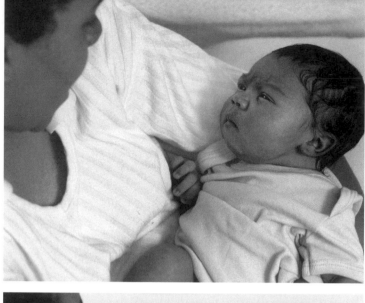

This baby girl is focusing on her mother's face.

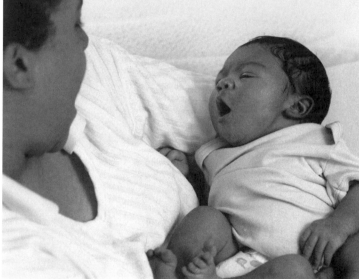

She widens her mouth in imitation of her mother.

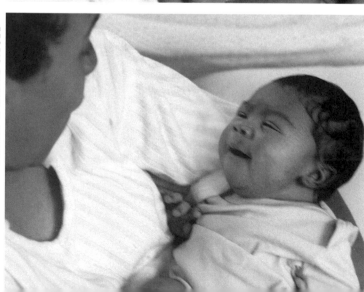

Sharing the pleasure of their dialogue

feelings related to the emotions they are imitating. Perhaps an innate ability in human infants to link what they see with what they sense in their own faces, along with natural mobility and activity of their features, account for the capacity of newborns to produce a broad range of facial expressions. As babies become older, their faces show expressions commonly shared by their particular family and culture to express genuine emotions. It is not uncommon to recognize an expression on your infant's face that reminds you of someone in the family.

During the entire time the baby is beginning to find himself in his mother's face, the mother herself is making many adjustments to the infant's face. Mothers-to-be often dream of their baby, and near the end of pregnancy will begin to develop a particular mental image of the infant. At the earliest moment of acquaintance after birth, mothers begin to replace the imagined baby with their real baby. Not only is there likely to be a marked difference between the expected and the real facial features, but the activity and behavior of the baby may also differ from the mother's expectations.

Intricacies of the relationship between mother and infant have been much illuminated by the perceptive observations of D. W. Winnicott, the renowned British pediatrician and psychoanalyst. He observed that mothers are a mirror for their babies and spend much time in the first months of life imitating their infants. He commented on this mirror role of the mother: "What does the baby see when he or she looks at the mother's face? I am suggesting that, ordi-narily, what the baby sees is himself or herself. In other words, the mother is looking at the baby and what she looks like is related to what she sees there. All this is too easily taken for granted. I am asking that this which is naturally done well by mothers who are caring for their babies shall not be taken for granted!" (D. W. Winnicott, *Playing and Reality*). Thus the mother and infant imitate each other. This process of the mother's pacing herself to her infant becomes especially important as the infant is beginning to discover his own being or boundaries.

The photos on the following pages show a short (30–45 seconds) emotional exchange between a nine-day-old infant and his sensitive grandfather. They illustrate an exciting interaction enabled by the grandfather's thoughtful pacing.

Babies appear to become more responsive when adults gently follow or imitate them rather than stimulate or lead them. Once a person has a well-integrated sense of self or personhood, he is likely to become upset if imitated. However, an infant's self is incompletely formed; the boundaries between the infant and others are not clear to him. Imitation of the infant's actions aids the process of self-discovery. After periods of active responding, babies tend to quiet down or turn off for a while, perhaps to rest, since too much play, either imitation or stimulation, tires them. Infants need frequent rest periods during and after interactions with their parents. This mutual mirroring is yet another way in which infants learn about how to act in their family.

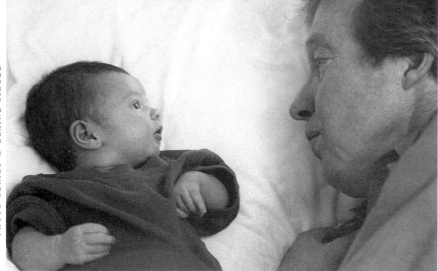

1 A 9-day-old baby and his grandfather have discovered each other. They begin a playful interaction while they look eye to eye.

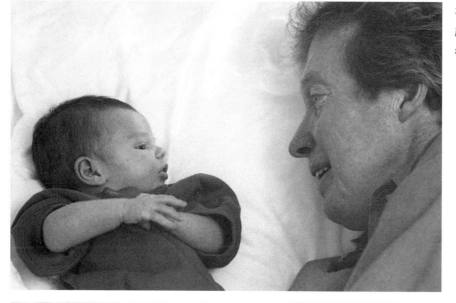

2 He observes grandfather's mouth and sees the mouth open.

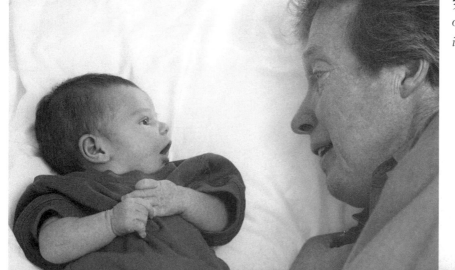

3 The baby then opens his mouth, imitating grandfather.

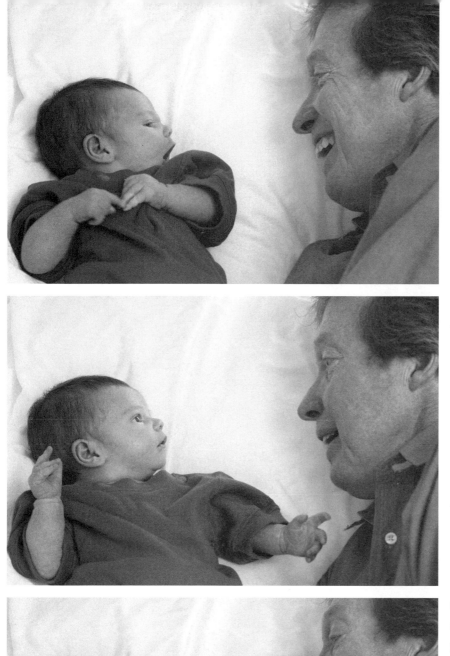

4 *Grandfather is delighted.*

5 *The infant again looks eye to eye.*

6 *The infant now reaches for the grandfather's mouth, where the game is being played.*

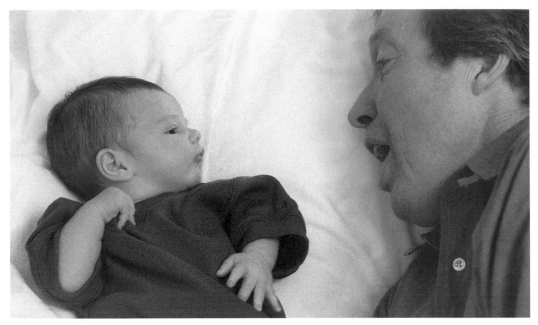

7   *The grandfather continues to play by opening his mouth wider, which the baby observes.*

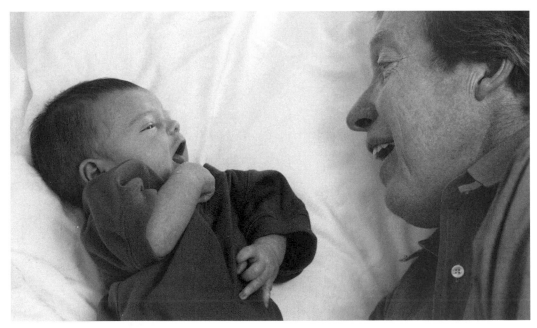

8   *With great energy he follows and opens his mouth widely.*

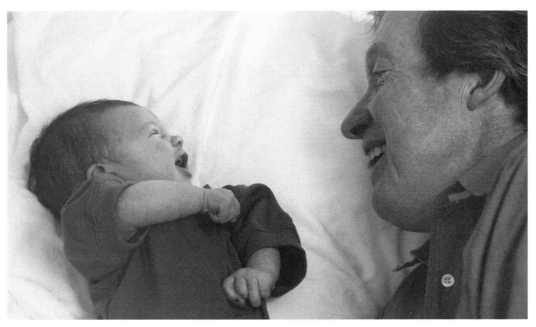

9 *Both take great delight in this joyful exchange. The baby throws his head back and opens his mouth even a bit wider.*

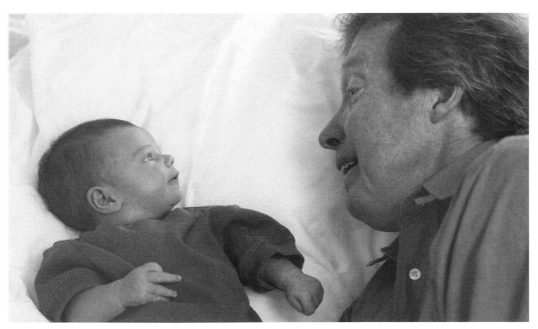

10 *Grandfather raises his eyebrows, and the baby follows with his eyes.*

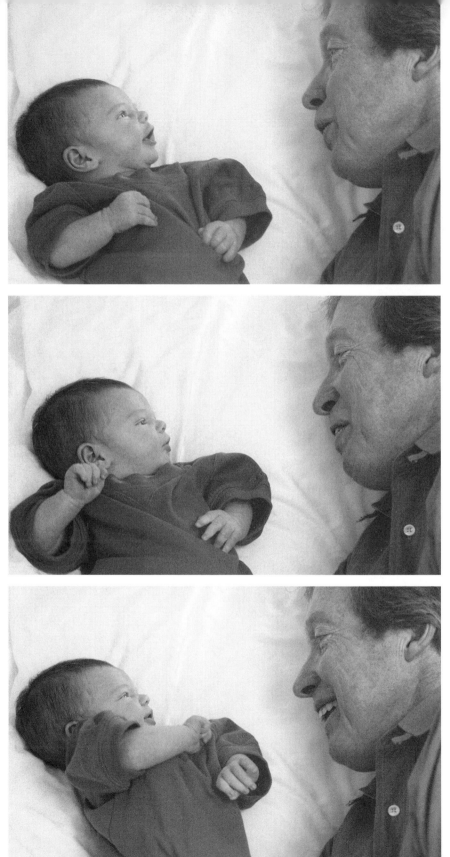

11 *Now grandfather switches to puckering his lips.*

12 *The baby focuses on the mouth and imitates the puckering.*

13 *They are both so pleased by this emotional engagement.*

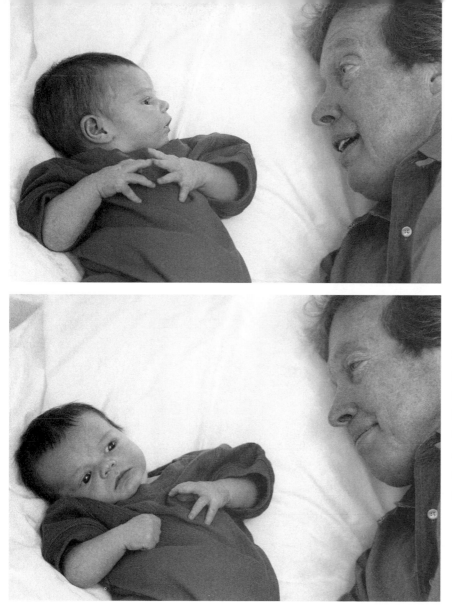

14 *The baby becomes serious and quiets down.*

15 *The grandfather paces himself to the baby, allowing him to turn away and rest, which is so important. All infants need frequent rest periods after intense interaction.*

It is not deliberate, self-conscious activity, but takes place at an almost unaware level of consciousness. We describe the process only because it is fun to know what is going on, not because either parent or baby needs to be coached; it comes naturally.

As parents spend time getting to know their baby, they gradually learn to put themselves in their infant's place. When they do, the signals the baby sends out to make his needs known or to elicit a response become increasingly clear. Within us all are amazing inborn systems for communicating, nurturing, and surviving.

THE NEWLY ADOPTED BABY

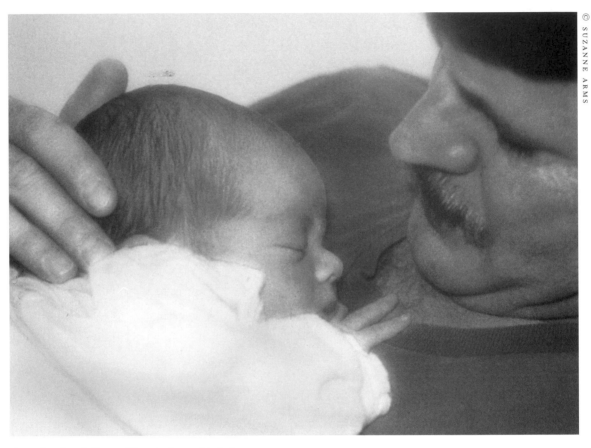

An adoptive father getting to know his baby

Parents and infants who find each other through adoption often travel a difficult road to make that connection. Our focus in this chapter is on the early adjustments of infants and their adoptive parents. Because not all babies are adopted as newborns, these adjustments are often made later. It is at that moment that both baby and parent can be said to be "newly born."

Adoptive parents must face complex issues and emotions in making the decision to adopt. By the time they have jumped through all the hoops required to prepare for adoption, parents can be left with a mixture of hope and great excitement, but also with some trepidation when that call finally comes to say, "You have a baby!" For some, simply hearing about an infant or receiving a picture generates an immediate rush of feelings. One mother said, "I knew she was mine the minute I saw her picture." Another mother remembered, "I fell in love with him when I held him in my arms for the first time." For others, the feelings grow more gradually after having the baby at home and taking care of her.

Interference that hinders adoptive mothers and fathers from learning their baby's signals can be similar to that experienced by any new parent: hospital routines that separate mothers from their new infants, problems with the baby's health, or, in the case of some domestic

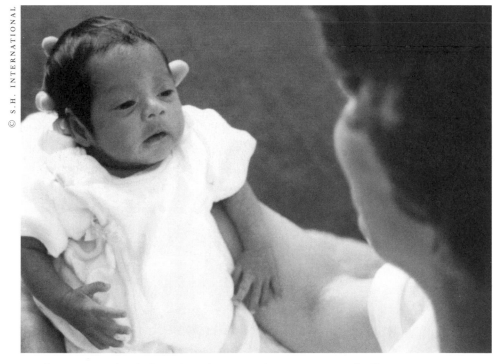

Mother enjoying her baby, adopted in Latin America, one week old

or international adoption regulations, weeks or months of residence in the birth mother's state or country before the baby can be moved to the new family. However, in most situations, parents cut through this interference and begin to learn about their baby.

One mother, who adopted in another state, described every detail of her first meeting with her baby daughter. This mother was very fortunate to be with her baby right from birth. "I saw her when she was fifteen minutes old. I was in a hospital gown, and after the baby was checked and her birth mother had the time she wanted, she was placed in my arms. She was quiet and peaceful. I held her continuously for the next two hours. She was very alert and aware. We looked eye to eye. I remember being so overwhelmed I was crying. My husband was taking pictures. We had a special quiet time together. I felt somewhat tentative. I wasn't sure how to hold her or exactly what I should do. She was my first baby. I wanted to take care of her in the best way. I felt an instantaneous attachment to her. I had been fearful that maybe I wouldn't attach to her. This was so contrary to my fears. I was instantly entranced by my baby; she was beautiful. She locked onto my eyes; she made a connection to me; it was like she was coming into my soul. I fell in love with her. I wanted to be with her and not leave her for a moment. In our situation the birth mother wanted to leave the hospital and return to her own home after a few hours. Very thoughtful nurses allowed me to stay on the maternity floor with our daughter, and I spent the night with her at my side. Like any new mother, I needed the help and support.

"After twenty-four to forty-eight hours, I had a feel of her in my arms. I could get her settled; I remember the delight I felt in making sounds with her. I would rock her, listen to music, and communicate with little sounds. Within a short time, I knew what upset her. Later, we had a bout with newborn colic. That was hard. I tried every trick of the trade. We got through that finally.

"That opportunity to bond right from the beginning was so important and valuable. I got to know her by having her with me, taking her everywhere, seeing how she reacted to different circumstances, what she could handle or not. You meet the baby's needs; you are her mother. The baby learns from you as you learn from her."

This baby's adoptive father remembers that he felt closer to her after a few days. It took him a while to figure out her signals, to feel at ease with caretaking. He relied on his wife and on the other experienced women around. Once they were in their own home, he jumped in eagerly with shared parenting. He was worried about making mistakes for about the first three months, but he felt more and more confident as time went on.

Not all adoptions start this early in the infant's life or go so smoothly. These parents benefited from the plans they made before the birth of the baby. They had developed a good

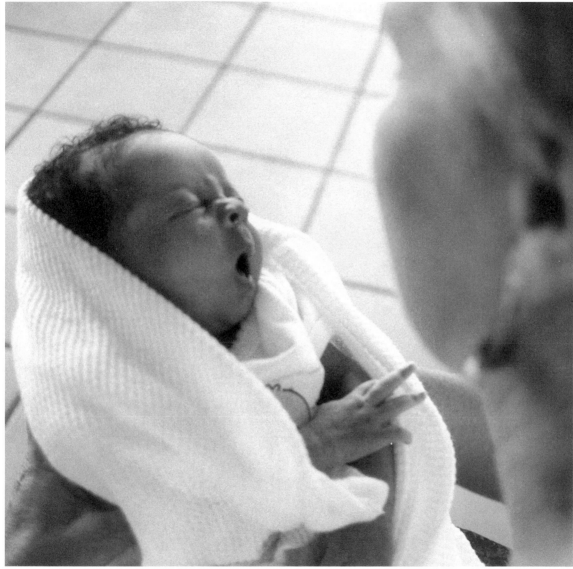

Mother learning the signals of her newly adopted baby

working relationship with the birth mother. They were especially fortunate that the hospital personnel understood who they were and appreciated the needs of the adoptive family as well as being sensitive to the birth mother.

Although difficulties arise in a small percentage of adoptions, they are far less common than the sensational stories in the press sometimes suggest. One father said to us, "Jump in, be optimistic, don't be afraid to treat the child as your own. If you're fearful, you won't engage, and some of the richness of the early period may be lost or not experienced fully."

When the couple described earlier adopted a second child, the hospital did not permit the parents to hold the baby even though he was screaming and the birth mother had completed her time with him. The adoptive mother recalled being terribly upset. Only the next day, after somebody intervened, was she allowed to hold her baby. The nursery kept the infant for a few days because of some minor problem. The adoptive mother remembers feeling exhausted and excluded and taking a little longer to feel the baby was hers: "It was more gradual. I remember wondering when it would occur. And now they are absolutely equal to me. He's a calm, easy, mellow baby. They are such different personalities, and it was not long before I realized that I felt like an experienced mother." The adoptive father also felt more seasoned with the second baby and handled the adoption with less anxiety about the legal process. He was aware, however, that it took him a little more time to feel hooked with his son, most likely because he missed the first week of his baby's life as he was, unavoidably, across the country.

For many families the adoption comes later, after a baby has a history of her own, and getting to know one another may take a little longer. A baby adopted after a few months may learn quickly to respond with smiles and gurgles to her new family, but be wary of initiating physical contact, such as cuddling or holding on, even when being held by her parents. If parents realize how disruptive it must be for a baby to go through a change of caretaker in the early months of life, they will soon find ways of comforting their baby; for instance, she may like to be held tightly when she is upset. Most babies will gradually begin to relax and to enjoy bath time, infant massage, and other infant games that involve human touch.

Many adoptive parents go to great lengths to maintain contact with the birth parent or to have photographs, letters, and even baby clothes or items that came with the infant as a way to keep a connection with the baby's roots. These will be treasured and will be helpful later to provide the child as complete a story as possible of her life. Parents who share this history with their child in an appropriate fashion as the child grows have an easier time integrating the adoption experience into a coherent life story for the child.

One mother described how, from a very early age, she told her adopted baby boy in a very simple manner all about his birth story and how

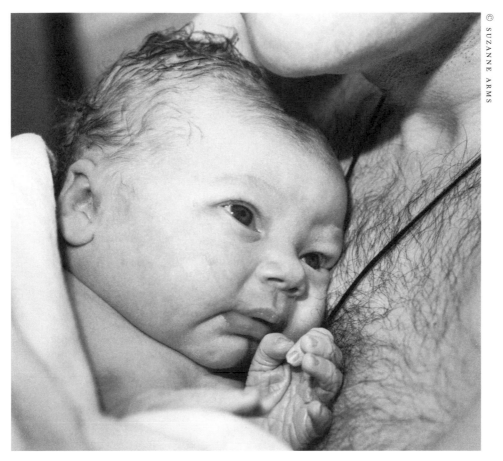

Newborn enjoying the closeness and warmth of skin-to-skin contact

he joined their family. As a toddler, he wanted to hear the story over and over, and this family found it very easy to have open discussions and answer any question he might have as he grew. The mother said, "He knew he was adopted right from the beginning, even though he may not have known what the word meant. I did not want it blurted out at a later age or for him to hear it from any other source. He also knew

that for me he was a miracle and that in all the world we found our way to each other." And she would often say to him, "We are a family forever."

One of the major tasks of any parent—adoptive or birth parent—is to learn the signals the baby is sending. Adoptive parents have found a number of simple ways to begin to feel a part of their new infant's life. Several mothers and fathers have commented how valuable it is to have skin-to-skin contact over some period of time. They and their babies find this mutually pleasing. This allows infant and parent to take each other in through a number of sensory experiences: smell, touch, temperature, sound, and so on.

All infants learn about their world through the many senses discussed in this book. Adoptive parents can give reassuring messages to their infants through holding, eye-to-eye contact, talking and singing to them, carrying them close in cloth carriers. If a child seems distant, perhaps not able fully to trust and more vulnerable because of her life experience before the adoption, the adoptive mother and father can pace themselves to her level of comfort, all the while providing steady form of love and connection. The baby often takes this in at a subliminal level and gradually begins to trust.

Techniques are also available to enable a mother to breast-feed even if she has never given birth. She can place a small bag of formula on her shoulder with a fine tube leading to her nipple, and as the baby sucks every two and a half to four hours her breast is stimulated by the infant's suckling, via her pituitary gland, to produce an increasing amount of milk. The supply of milk typically increases in three or four days, but it takes up to two weeks to obtain a satisfactory output. Through this technique the mother can usually meet up to 70 to 90 percent of the infant's needs. Some mothers have found that combining relaxation exercise with visualizing or imagining their milk flowing freely has resulted in a remarkable increase in their milk supply.

In our experience, many adoptive mothers take from two to six months off from work to become acquainted with their baby and help both the baby and themselves become adjusted to their new family life. Fathers often stay home as well for some of this time. This is a terribly important time for parents and baby. Even though the mother has not given birth, she will experience many or most of the emotional changes that a new baby brings: excitement, insecurity, caregiving, exhaustion, with nights and days rolled into one. Working out coparenting roles and finding helpful, nurturing support from other people are essential. Keeping a quiet private time, lowering demands on oneself, and limiting visitors are also important. A new child is a major transition for both parents and needs to be respected as such.

A significant number of children join their adoptive families after a period of being cared for by foster parents or being in a short-term institutional setting. The longer the time before the child joins a permanent family, the longer the time the child will need to adjust and adapt to the caretaking practices of the adoptive family. The baby or child must first mourn the loss of previous family or caretakers. It can be difficult for parents not to feel rejected or disappointed if the attachment is not immediate. The gradual adaptation will require patience, time, and sensitivity to the child's needs and signals.

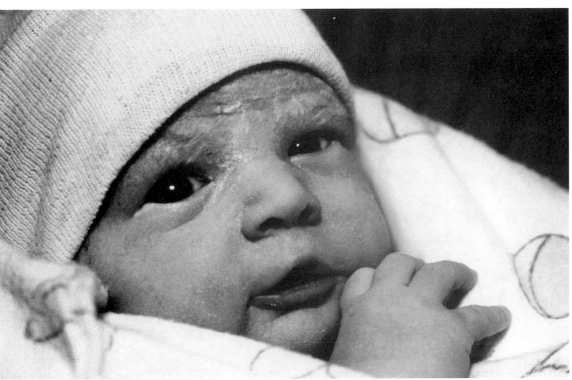

Dressed for the first time, this hour-old boy gazes forth at his new world.

This early loss may be evidenced by sadness or bouts of unexplained crying or by responses of protest, rage, or despair. Some level of loss can also be experienced by an infant adopted at or soon after birth. Because the prenatal life of the infant carries experiences that are registered deep in the psyche and the first moments after birth make a deep impression, there cannot be a disconnection from a birth mother without an experience of loss. Premature infants and newborns separated for medical reasons from their birth mothers suffer a similar pain of separation.

They will need the same empathic, patient care to allow for a gradual adjustment and growing feeling of security.

Adoptive parents may have to work extra hard to provide the consistent care and emotional love and energy that gives a feeling of secure attachment to their infant. Sometimes, noticing unexplained sadness, adoptive mothers may gently acknowledge the loss, with or without words. Given time, patience, and sensitive reading of the baby's signals, the foundation for a secure attachment will be laid. However, when

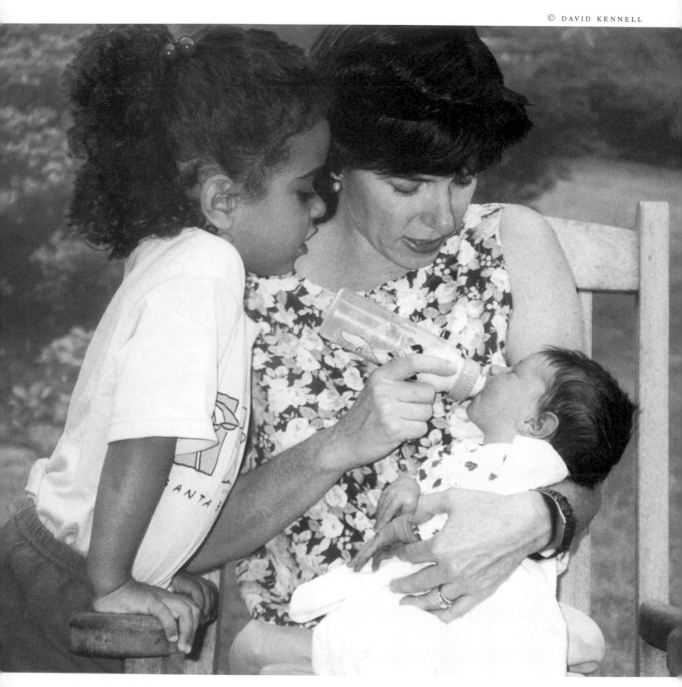

An adopted three-year-old watches her new adopted brother.

there has been severe deprivation or inadequate care before the adoption, adoptive parents may need extra help to mend the psychological and emotional damage the child has sustained.

Each parent brings a lifetime of expectations to adoption. One father, preparing for a trans-racial adoption, observed the many different children on the bus as he went to work each morning. He could not visualize himself as a father of any these children whose race differed from his own. He was therefore totally surprised by his own feelings when he saw his new baby for the first time. She was the most beautiful baby he had ever seen, and he felt she was his from the very first moment. This little girl was from another culture, racial group, and country. Parents for whom the adoption brings a first child cannot predict how they will feel when their infant crawls under their chin, holds on tightly, and nestles peacefully.

Many parents who adopt children across racial lines continue to respect the child's heritage. For instance, white families may arrange special Chinese language lessons for their Chinese-born children or ask for instruction in the proper care of their African American baby's hair and skin.

Many early challenges are the same in both adoptive and nonadoptive families. Babies may have colic, different temperaments, or more intense needs than other family members. All parents have the task of figuring out how to handle these difficulties. Adoption is only one of the many unknowns that influence every child's later adjustment. Obviously, the parenting skills

of open communication, comfort with touch, holding, loving, responsive interactions, consistent but warm boundary setting, and flexible and caring relationships between parents can enhance the family's growth and adjustment. In the early months, as we have pointed out, figuring out the baby's signals, often through trial and error, is the first crucial task.

One of the questions that many adoptive parents ask themselves is, "Am I bonded to my baby?" This concern arises because parents have heard that early contact is necessary to develop a close bond with their infant. To keep these fears in perspective, it is helpful to realize that once parents have met their new baby, feeling love for the baby occurs on about the same timetable for both adoptive and birth parents. In an informal survey, two-thirds of both groups of mothers (adoptive and birth) reported feeling love for their baby at the first contact with the infant or before (either during pregnancy or from knowledge or a picture of the baby that was coming to them). But new parenthood brings a wide range of feelings. Although all new parents experience thrilled, happy, and ecstatic feelings, they may also feel relief, surprise, worries about their baby, or sadness. In other words, being a first-time parent, whether by birth or adoption, evokes a variety of feelings, and although many parents feel attached to their baby at first contact, many others find it takes a week or longer to feel the baby is theirs.

It is interesting to note that when the birth mother or woman who is not the mother spend an hour with a baby they will be equally able to

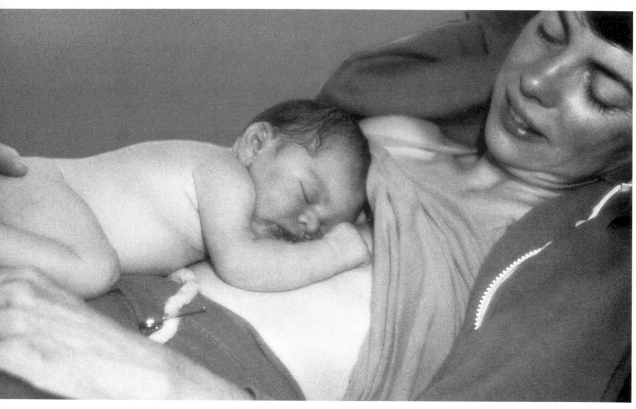

An adoptive mother getting to know her baby in the first hours of life

identify that infant's undershirt from two others. (The shirts are put in a plastic bag so that sight is not involved.)

Although early contact for both birth and adoptive parents is valuable for them and their baby, developing emotional ties to the baby is dependent on many other factors as well. Emotional readiness for a baby opens the hearts and minds of expectant parents for the long period of adjustment, concern, and joy ahead. First-time adoptive parents especially may benefit from a class or parents' group that provides information about infant-care skills, what changes may occur in the marital relationship, and the common emotional highs and lows that come with every new infant.

THE NEWBORN FAMILY

10

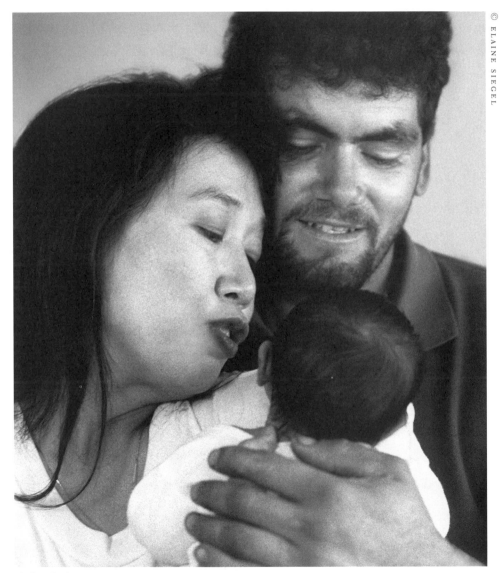

A family begins.

© ELAINE SIEGEL

After the months of waiting and preparing and the hours of birthing, the baby has finally arrived, bringing feelings of relief, happiness, wonder, and disbelief. Mothers are already somewhat familiar with the baby whom they carried, and fathers have hope mixed with anxiety and anticipation. Now the baby is in their arms, in their family, and begins to find a way into their hearts.

A myriad of sensory, immunological, hormonal, physiological, and behavioral events built into both the parents and the baby begin to emerge in this early period of attaching to each other. These experiences enable parents to take in their baby, to learn their baby's signals, and to meet his needs appropriately. The incredible attributes that we have seen in the newborn have a major purpose. They prepare the baby for interaction with his family and for life in the world.

Nature also activates each member of the family in unique ways to receive the baby. When holding their infant for the first time, mothers almost invariably explore him in a particular order. They initially touch the infant's arms and legs with their fingertips in a fashion somewhat similar to a cook's testing a cake to see if it is finished. After a few minutes, sometimes after just a few seconds, many mothers proceed to massage, touch, and stroke their infant's body. Fathers start the process of getting to know their baby in similar ways.

At this very early time, parents have a special interest in the infant's eyes and unconsciously try to align their faces on the same parallel plane of rotation as their infant's face. This is called the *en face*, or face-to-face, position. We have observed this not only with parents who are getting to know their full-term babies, but also with mothers and fathers of premature babies. Mothers have to tilt their heads a great deal to move themselves into the *en face* position with a premature infant who is in the hospital nursery.

These tentative early greetings are accompanied by a tide of new feelings. During the first hour of life, as already noted, there is an extended period of quiet alertness in the newborn infant. The infant looks at his mother's face, follows and responds to her voice. Mothers and fathers often express an unusual sense of excitement when they begin to make contact with their baby. Many mothers report feeling warmly close to their infant after the infant has looked at them, acknowledging the importance of relating to the baby through eye contact. More than one mother has said, "Open your eyes. Oh, come on, open your eyes. If you open your eyes, I'll know you're mine."

Illustrating the subtle and astonishing processes under way in the first hour of life is a recent observation that when a mother has her infant with her for just one hour after birth, she unconsciously learns to identify her baby from other babies by two primary senses, smell and touch. When blindfolded and asked ten hours later to pick out her baby's undershirt from three undershirts or the back of her baby's hand from others, she can easily recognize her own infant. Within another day, most mothers can

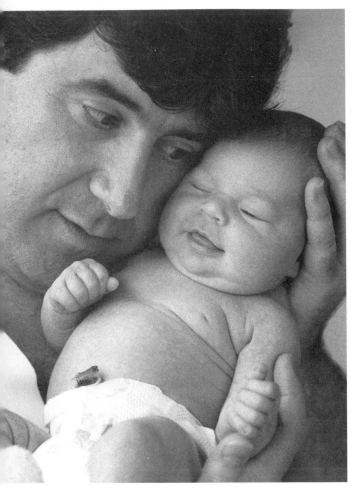 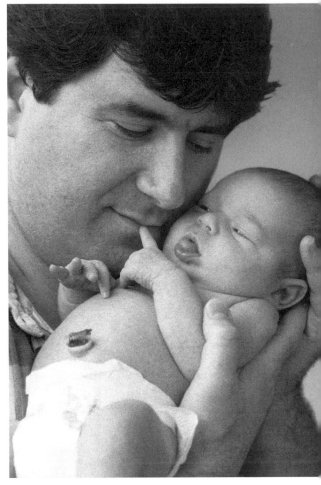

Father enjoying his infant daughter

also recognize their own baby from a photograph or from his cry in comparison with those of two other newborns.

In the first week or so, there are rapidly changing emotions for both mother and father and bodily changes for the mother. As the mother's body and hormones begin to return to a prebirth state, periods of letdown or blues may occur at the same time as she is becoming accustomed to her newborn. Fathers also experience shifting emotions, from the sense of enormous capability of having produced their infant to immense feelings of responsibility. Fathers and mothers often experience differing needs. At this time, fathers are both engrossed in and tentative with the newborn, and mothers are both exhausted and enamored. Both parents do better if they can talk together about these feelings. This is a period of learning about not only the baby's needs, but each other's.

These early periods together are especially rewarding and important for another reason. Some women fear that they might give birth to an infant who is not perfect. They cannot believe that they are good enough to produce a completely normal infant. For these mothers, as well as for fathers with similar fears, these early private times together replace some of the anxieties they feel at birth with a sense of grateful wonder.

Parents who miss these early periods with their infant or do not feel an immediate love for their baby sometimes believe that they cannot be bonded or attached to their baby in a normal fashion or that something is lost in their future relationship with the baby. As we saw in Chapter 9, such doubts are unfounded. Many people misunderstand the process of bonding and give too literal a meaning to the word *bonding*, as though it were a mechanical process — the "epoxy model." Attachment to their infant occurs at different times for different people. For many parents, it happens during the first moments or a day or two after birth; for others, it does not occur until they are home from the hospital and taking care of their infant for the first time alone.

One mother described her feelings in this way: "My husband, particularly after we had the first visit with the baby, said, 'He's ours, I know he's ours, and I love him very much.' I knew I loved him, but it took me a little bit longer to realize that this baby was ours. Until he was in our home and I was taking care of him I didn't feel he was mine."

Another couple had a different experience. The mother commented, "There was a rush of feelings after delivery, you could hear him and he was real. I could still see the connection between him and me. He was so beautiful and he was okay." This woman's husband said, "I was surprised at how he looked. I really hadn't any mental image of what he would look like. It was just like a lump in her belly and here it was a person."

Dr. Winnicott's description of primary maternal preoccupation is helpful in understanding this period of life for the mother. "It is a state of heightened sensitivity that lasts for a few weeks after the birth . . . [which] provides a setting for the infant's individuality to make itself evident, for the developmental tendencies to start to unfold, and for the infant to become the owner of the sensations that are appropriate to this early phase of life. A mother who is in this state can feel herself into her infant's place" (Winnicott 1958).

As we saw in the previous chapters, an amazing mutuality pervades the relationship between mother and newborn. The mother appears to be unusually receptive to learning about and perceiving her infant through all her senses. The infant's talents, abilities, and wide range of senses are each matched by parallel sensitivities and alertness on the part of the mother. There is a mutual interest in eye-to-eye contact. A mother's use of a high-pitched voice in talking to her infant coincides with the infant's attraction to speech in the high-frequency range. The timing of speech stimulates both parent and infant to move to its rhythm. An infant's cry will stimulate milk production. As we noted earlier, during bottle or breast-feeding, the distance between the parent and the infant's eyes is about eight to ten inches, an optimum distance for a newborn to see his mother or his father.

Not only does breast milk transmit defenses against infection to the baby, but the infant's sucking action causes hormones to be produced in the mother that help return her uterus to its former shape. In addition, when the infant suckles from the breast, special cells in both the mother's and infant's brains secrete oxytocin (also known as the "cuddle hormone") into the brain. Increased brain oxytocin results in slight sleepiness, mild euphoria, a raised threshold for pain and, most appropriately, increased love for the baby. We have wondered whether this frequent increase of the cuddle hormone in the baby's brain with each feeding also helps build the infant's attraction for his mother.

All the baby's senses are especially alert as well. For example, when a baby is feeding and parents start to talk, the baby stops sucking or changes his sucking rate as he tries to listen. These pauses occur mainly on hearing the mother's voice, not other sounds. The baby rewards the mother for fondling, kissing, cuddling, and prolonged gazing by looking into her eyes, smiling, turning to her voice, and quieting to her touch. Mother and infant, especially suited to each other physiologically, hormonally, and emotionally, respond to each other on a number of sensory and social levels that serve to lock the pair together.

Many parents look back on this early time of closeness as deeply joyful and meaningful. The more time parents can spend with their infant in the first few days, the better they will understand their baby and be able to meet his needs. Once they are at home, fathers also benefit greatly by having their own private time with their infant. When a father is asked to play with his infant in the first hours and to establish eye-to-eye contact with the baby, he spends considerably more time with the baby in the first three months than do fathers who don't have this experience. Fathers have their own style of nurturing their baby and derive great pleasure from these early hours and days. Videotapes show that fathers

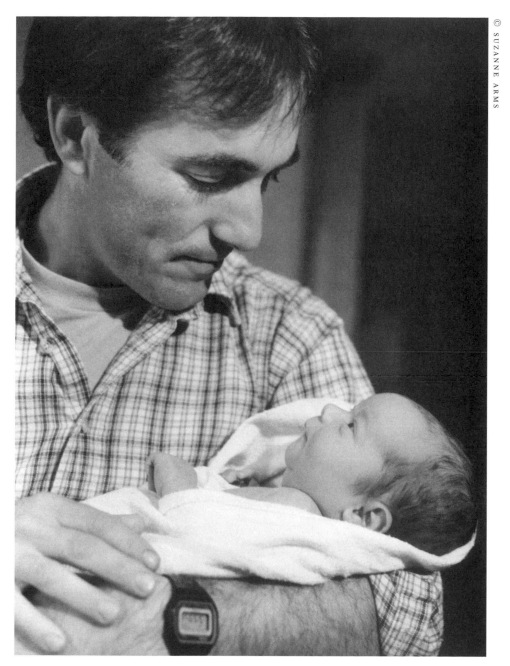

A father holds his newborn baby.

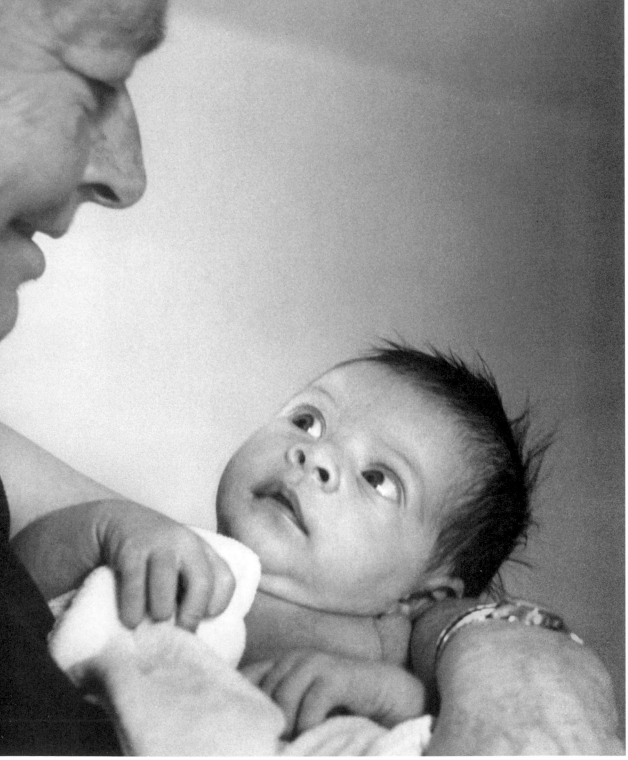

Infant girl meeting her grandmother

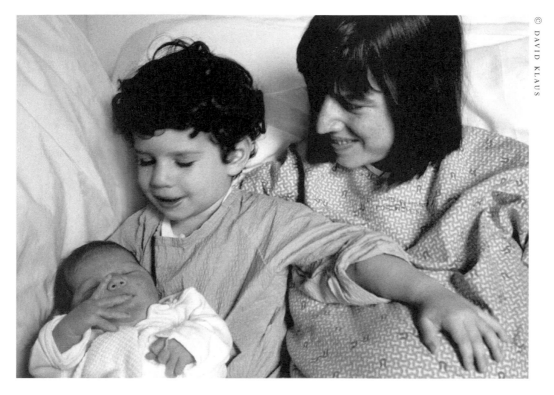

tend to be more active and playful with their infant than are mothers and that babies soon learn to anticipate the fun. Grandparents need little encouragement to enjoy a new baby, and early contact helps them feel close as well.

Once the infant is home, the father has a much easier time taking care of him and getting to know him. One father's own words describe what can happen: "He's so communicative. His typical pattern is to wake up and nurse a bit, and then I'll take him in and change him, and he's good on the changing table. By then, he's bright-eyed and alert and he just really takes in everything around him, and he'll focus on you and you get really great eye contact with him. He responds to your talking, and if he fusses a little

bit, I pick him up; he always calms down. He's a very responsive kid. I don't think I ever expected that at so young an age."

Siblings, too, can benefit from the earliest possible contact with the newborn. Since young children have a different concept of time than do adults, they sometimes believe they have been abandoned for an extended period when they have actually been separated from their mother for only a couple of days. This short separation commonly results in temper tantrums, sleep disturbances, and eating problems for the child. It is recommended that siblings visit their mother daily. Parents sometimes doubt whether a sibling should come to the hospital because little children often cry when

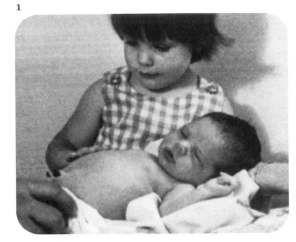

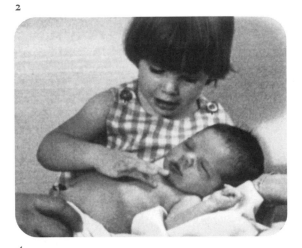

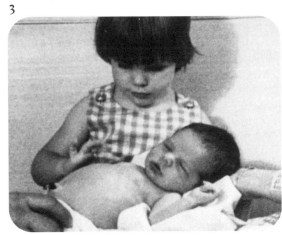

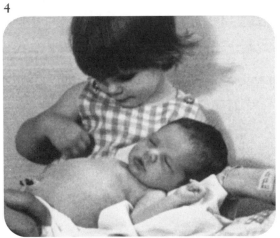

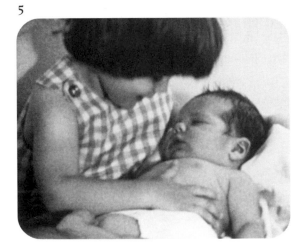

These video shots show a young girl holding her sister for the first time.

1 *She touches the baby's abdomen.*

2 *She touches one nipple.*

3 *She now examines her sister's other nipple.*

4 *She compares the baby with herself.*

5 *She then moves closer and hugs her sister.*

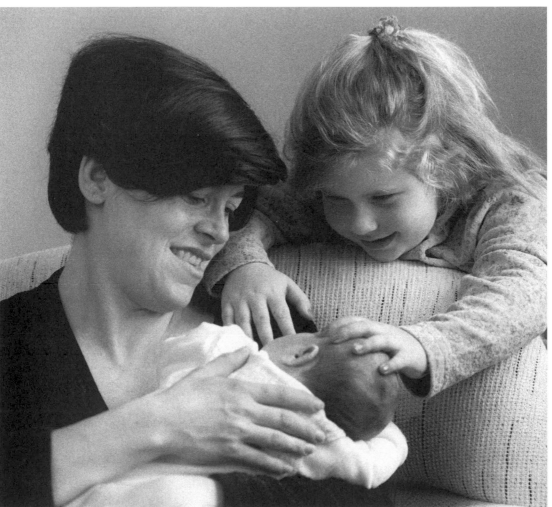

Getting to know the new member of the family

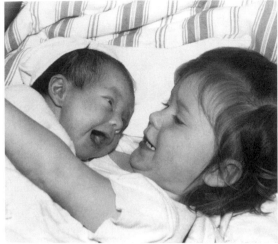

9-hour-old infant with her sister

the visit is over. However, the benefits far out-weigh the relatively short-lived distress that occurs when the young child must leave. It is important to remember that the young siblings are coming in to see their mother first and fore-most and only secondarily to see the infant. Mothers should take a little time to play alone with the sibling before focusing on the baby.

When the older sibling has been more involved with the newborn from the start, the homecoming is often less fraught with anxieties. As babies get older, they begin to show a special fascination for other children, for someone clearly closer to their own size than are adults. The awestruck gaze of a baby can help win over the most skeptical older brother or sister.

This is only the beginning in the complex

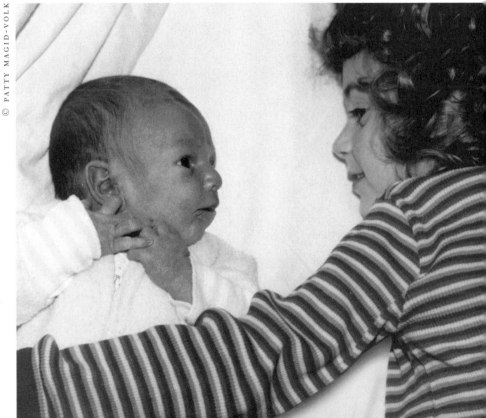

*Meeting a new brother
for the first time*

104

process by which families become attached to their newborn infant. Mothers and fathers can expect an ever-increasing range of emotions as the infant grows. A Mayan Indian saying tells us: "In the baby lies the future of the world. The mother must hold him close so he will know the world is his. The father must take him to the highest hill so he can see what his world is like."

As the newborn grows, parents change and grow. Falling in love with a baby changes how we respond not only to the baby, but to our whole world. The observant, patient nurturing becomes so rewarding that parents rearrange their lives. As the baby responds in ever more subtle ways, a profound relationship builds. The more sensitive they are to the clues of the infant, the easier it will be to respond to him. Babies begin to trust these responses, and parents begin truly to believe they are the right parents for their baby. Babies in this loving circle adapt to the family routine and gradually develop the foundations of a secure attachment.

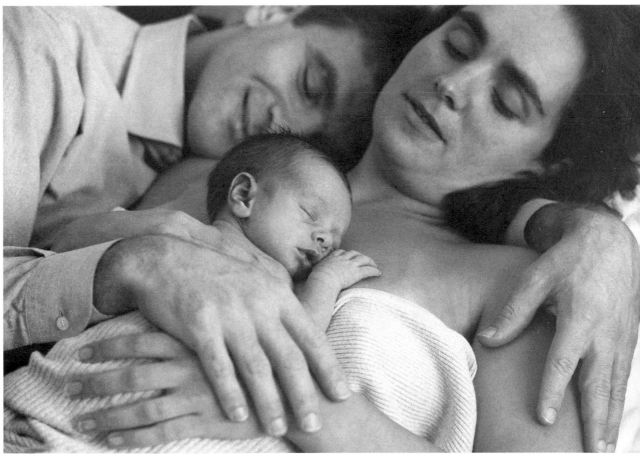

A very new family resting together

REFERENCES

CHAPTER 1

Ando, Y., and Hattori, H. Effects of noise on sleep of babies. *Journal of the Acoustical Society of America* 62(1): 199–204, 177.

Birnholz, J. C., and Benacerraf, B. R. The development of human fetal hearing. *Science* 222: 516–518, 1983.

Birnholz, J. C., and Farrell, E. E. Ultrasound images of human fetal development. *American Scientist* 72: 608–614, 1984.

deVries, J. I. P., Visser, G. H. A., and Prechtl, H. F. R. The emergence of fetal behavior: 3. Individual differences and consistencies. *Early Human Development* 16: 85–103, 1988.

Mirmiran, M., and Kok, J. H. Circadian rhythms in early human development. *Early Human Development* 26: 121–128, 1991.

Nathanielsz, M. *Life before birth and a time to be born.* Ithaca, N. Y.: Promethean Press, 1992.

Pillai, M., and James, D. Behavioral states in normal mature fetuses. *Archives of Pediatrics and Adolescent Medicine* 65: 39–43, 1990.

Prechtl, H. F. R. Prenatal motor development. In *Motor development in children: Aspects of coordination and control*, edited by M. G. Wade and H. T. A. Whiting, pp. 53–64. Dordrecht, Netherlands: Martinus Nijhoff Publishers, 1986.

Wisser, J., and Dirschedl, P. Embryonic heart rate in dated human embryos. *Early Human Development* 37: 107–115, 1994.

CHAPTER 2

Christensson, K. Fathers can effectively achieve heat conservation in healthy newborn infants. *Acta Paediatrica* 85: 1354–1360, 1996.

Christensson, K., Siles, C., Moreno, L. Belaustqua, A., de la Fuente, P. P., Lagercrantz, H., Puol, P., and Winberg, J. Temperature, metabolic adapta-tion and crying in healthy, full-term newborn babies cared for skin-to-skin or in a cot. *Acta Paediatrica* 81: 488–493, 1992.

Righard, L., and Alade, M. O. Effect of delivery routines on success of first breast-feed. *Lancet* 336: 1105–1107, 1990.

Schaal, B., Marlier, L., and Soussignon, R. Responsiveness to odour of amniotic fluid in the human neonate. *Biology of the Neonate* 67: 397–406, 1995.

Varendi, H., Porter, R. H., and Winberg, J. Does the newborn find the nipple by smell? *Lancet* 344: 989-990, 1994.

Varendi, H., Porter, R. H., and Winberg, J. Attractiveness of amniotic fluid odor: Evidence of prenatal olfactory learning? *Acta Paediatrica* 85: 1223–1227, 1996.

Widström, A. M., Ransjö-Arvidson, A. B., Christensson, K., Mathieson, A. S., Winberg, J., and Uvnäs-Moberg, K. Gastric suction in healthy newborn infants: Effects on circulation and developing feeding behavior. *Acta Paediatrica* 76: 566–572, 1987.

Widström, A. M., Wahlburg, W., Mathiesen, A. S., Enroth, P., Uvnäs-Moberg, K., Wernert, S., and Winberg, J. Short-term effects of early suckling and touch of the nipple on maternal behavior. *Early Human Development* 21: 153–163, 1990.

CHAPTER 3

Anders, T. F. Biological rhythms in development. *Psychosomatic Medicine* 44(1): 61–72, 1982.

Brazelton, T. B. Psychophysiologic reactions in the neonate: The value of observation of the neonate. *Journal of Pediatrics* 58: 508-312, 1961.

Brazelton, T. B. *Neonatal Behavioral Assessment Scale*, 3rd Edition. New York: Cambridge University Press, 1996.

Emde, R. N., Swedburg, J., and Suzuki, B. Human

wakefulness and biological rhythms after birth. *Archives of General Psychiatry* 32: 780–783, 1975.

Glotzbach, S. F., Edgar, D. M., Boeddiker, M., and Ariagno, R. L. Biological rhythmicity in normal infants during the first three months of life. *Pediatrics* 94: 483–488, 1994.

Prechtl, H. F. R. and O'Brien, M. J. Behavioral states of the full-term newborn: The emergence of a concept. In *Psychobiology of the human newborn*, edited by P. Stratton. New York: John Wiley & Sons, 1982.

Weinert, D., Sitka, V., Minors, D. S., and Waterhouse, J. M. The development of circadian rhythmicity in neonates. *Early Human Development* 36: 117–126, 1994.

Wolff, P. H. Observation on newborn infants. *Psychosomatic Medicine* 21: 110–118, 1959.

Wolff, P. H. The development of behavioral states and the expression of emotions in early infancy. In *A new proposal for investigation*. Chicago: University of Chicago Press, 1987.

CHAPTER 4

Braddick, O. Binocularity in infancy. *Eye* 10: 182–188, 1996.

Courage, M. L., and Adams, R. J. Infant peripheral vision: The development of monocular visual acuity in the first three months of post-natal life. *Vision Research* 36: 1207–1215, 1996.

Dougherty, T. M., and Haith, M. M. Infant expectations and reaction time as predictors of childhood speed of processing and IQ. *Developmental Psychology* 33: 146–155, 1997.

Fantz, R. L. The origin of form perception. *Scientific American* 204: 66–72, 1961.

——.Pattern vision in newborn infants. *Science* 140: 296–297, 1963.

——.Visual experience in infants: Decreased attention to familiar relative to novel ones. *Science* 146: 668–670, 1964.

Hainline, L., and Riddell, P. M. Binocular alignment and vergence in early infancy. *Vision Research* 35: 3229–3236, 1995.

Haith, M. M. Sensory and perceptual processes in early infancy. *Journal of Pediatrics* 109: 158–171, 1986.

Mehler, J., Dupoux, E. What infants know: The new cognitive science of early development. Cambridge, Mass: Blackwell, 1994.

Meltzoff, A. N., and Borton, R. W. Intermodal matching by human neonates. *Nature* 282: 403–404, 1979.

Pascalis, O., de Schonen, S., Morton, J., Deruelle, O., and Fabre-Grenet, M. Mother's face recognition by neonate: A replication and extension. *Infant Behavior and Development* 18: 79–86, 1995.

Walton, G. E., Bower, N. J. A., and Bower, T. G. R. Recognition of familiar forms by newborns. *Infant Behavior and Development* 15: 265–269, 1992.

CHAPTER 5

DeCasper, A. J., and Fifer, W. P. Of human bonding: Newborns prefer their mothers' voices. *Science* 208: 1174–1176, 1980.

DeCasper, A. J., Lecanuet, J. P., Busnel, M. C., Granier-Deferre, C., and Maugeais, R. Fetal reactions to recurrent maternal speech. *Infant Behavior and Development* 17: 159–164, 1994.

DeCasper, A. J., and Spence, M. J. Prenatal maternal speech influences newborns' perception of speech sounds. *Infant Behavior and Development* 9: 133–150, 1986.

DeCasper, A. J., and Spence, M. J. Auditory mediated behavior during the perinatal period: A cognitive view. In *Newborn attention: Biological constraints and the influence of experience*, edited by M. J. S. Weiss and P. R. Zelazo. Norwood, N.J.: Ablex, 1991.

Fernald, A. Intonation and communicative intent in mothers' speech to infants: Is the melody the message? Child Development 60: 1497–1510, 1989.

Fernald, A. Approval and disapproval: Infant responsiveness to vocal affect in familiar and unfamiliar languages. *Child Development* 64: 657–674, 1993.

Kuhl, P. K., Andruski, J. E., Chistovich, I. A., Chistovich, L. A., Kozhevnikova, E. V., Ryskina, V. L., Stolyarova, E. I., Sundberg, U., and Lacerda, F. Cross-language analysis of phonetic units in language addressed to infants. *Science* 277: 684–686, 1997.

Papousek, M., Bornstein, M. H., Nuzzo, C., Papousek, H., and Synames, D. Infant responses to prototypical melodic contours in parental speech. *Infant Behavior and Development* 13: 539–545, 1990.

CHAPTER 6

Acolet, D., Modi, N., Giannakoulopoulos, X., Bond, C., Weg, W., Clow, A., and Glover, V. Changes in plasma cortisol and catecholamine concentrations in response to massage in preterm infants. *Archives of Pediatrics and Adolescent Medicine* 68: 29–31, 1993.

Blass, E. Changing influences of sucrose and visual engagement in 2 to 12-week-old human infants: Implications for maternal face recognition. *Infant Behavior and Development* 20: 423–434, 1997.

Blass, E. M., and Hoffmeyer, L. B. Sucrose as an analgesic for newborn infants. *Pediatrics* 87: 215–218, 1991.

Field, T., Schanberg, S., Scafidi, F., Bauer, C. R., Garcia, R., Nystrom, J., and Kuhn, C. M. Tactile kinesthetic stimulation effects on preterm neonates. *Pediatrics* 77: 654–658, 1986.

MacFarlane, A. Olfaction in the development of social preferences in the human neonate. In *Parent-infant interaction*, edited by R. Porter and M. O'Connor, Ciba Foundation Symposium 33, Amsterdam: American Elsevier, 1975.

Mennella, A. Mother's milk: A medium for early flavor experiences. *Journal of Human Lactation* 11: 39–45, 1995.

Montagu, A. *Touching: The human significance of the skin.* New York: Columbia University Press, 1971.

Porter, R. H., Makin, J. W., Davis, L. B., and Christensson, K. Breast-fed infants respond to olfactory cues from their own mother and unfamiliar lactating females. *Infant Behavior and Development* 15: 85–93, 1992.

Schaal, B., Marlier, L., and Soussignon, R. Responsiveness to the odour of amniotic fluid in the human neonate. *Biology of the Neonate* 67: 397–406, 1995.

Varendi, H., Porter, R. H., and Winberg, J. Attractiveness of amniotic fluid odor: Evidence of prenatal olfactory learning. *Acta Paediatrica* 85: 1223–1227, 1996.

Winberg, J., and Porter, R. H. Olfaction and human neonatal behavior: Clinical implications. *Acta Paediatrica* 87: 6–10, 1998.

CHAPTER 7

Amiel-Tison, C., and Grenier, A. *Neurological assessment during the first year of life.* New York: Oxford University Press, 1986.

Bushnell, E. W., and Boudreau, J. P. Motor development and the mind: The potential role of motor abilities as a determinant of aspects of perceptual development. *Child Development* 64: 1005–1021, 1993.

Condon, W. S., and Sander, L. W. Neonate movement is synchronized with adult speech: Interactional participation and language acquisition. *Science* 183: 99–101, 1974.

Robertson, S. S. Intrinsic temporal patterning in the sponstaneous movement of awake neonates. *Child Development* 53: 1016–1021, 1982.

Robertson, S. S., Dierker, L. J., Sorokin, Y., and Rosen, M. G. Human fetal movement: Spontaneous oscillations near one cycle per minute. *Science* 218: 1327–1330, 1982.

Thoman, E. B., Ingersoll, E. W., and Acebo, C. Premature infants seek rhythmic stimulation and the experience facilitates neurobehavioral development. *Journal of Developmental Behavioral Pediatrics* 12: 11–18, 1991.

CHAPTER 8

Ekman, P., and Davidson, R. J., *The nature of emotion: Fundamental questions.* New York: Oxford University Press, 1994.

Field, T. M., Woodson, R., Greenberg, R., and Cohen,

D. Discrimination and imitation of facial expressions by infants. *Science* 218: 179–181, 1982.

Kaitz, M., Meschulach-Sarfaty, O., and Auerbach, J. A re-examination of newborns' ability to imitate facial expressions. *Developmental Psychology* 24: 3–7, 1988.

Maratos, O. Trends in the development of imitation in early infancy. In *Regressions in mental development,* edited by T. G. Bever. Hillsdale, NJ: Lawrence Erlbaum Associates, 1982.

Meltzoff, A. N. Towards a developmental cognitive science: Implications of cross-modal matching and imitation for the development of memory in infancy. *Annals of the New York Academy of Sciences* 608: 1–37, 1990.

Meltzoff, A. N. and Moore, M. K. Newborn infants imitate adult facial gestures. *Child Development* 54: 702–709, 1983.

Sia, F., and Bushness, I. W. R. The perception of faces in different poses by one-month-olds. *Journal of Developmental Psychology* 6: 35–41, 1988.

Termini, N. T., and Izard, C. E. Infants' responses to their mothers' expressions of joy and sadness. *Developmental Psychology* 24: 223–229, 1988.

Winnicott, D. W. *Playing and reality.* London: Tavistock Publications, 1971.

CHAPTER 9

Arms, S. *Adoption, a handful of hope.* Berkeley, Calif.: Celestial Arts, 1983.

Hostetter, M., Iverson, S., and Thomas, W. Medical evaluation of internationally adopted children. *New England Journal of Medicine* 325: 479–485, 1991.

Kaitz, M., and Eidelman, A. I. Smell recognition of newborns by women who are not mothers. *Chemical Senses* 17: 225–229, 1992.

Rosenberg, E. *The adoption life cycle: The children and their families through the years.* New York: The Free Press/Macmillan, 1993.

Tizard, B. *Adoption: A second chance.* London: Open Books, 1977.

Verrier, N. N. *The primal wound: Understanding the adopted chld.* Baltimore: Gatyeway Press, 1993.

CHAPTER 10

Brazelton, T. B., and Cramer, B. G. *The earliest relationship.* Cambridge, Mass.: Perseus Books, 1990.

Eidelman, A., and Kaitz, M. Olfactory recognition: A genetic or learned capacity? *Journal of Developmental and Behavioral Pediatrics* 13: 126–127, 1992.

Kaitz, M., Good, A., Rokem, A. M., and Eidelman, A. I. Mothers' recognition of their newborns by olfactory cues. *Developmental Psychology* 20: 587–591, 1987.

Kaitz, M. Lapidot, P., and Bronner, R. Parturient women can recognize their infants by touch. *Developmental Psychology* 28: 35–39, 1992.

Kaitz, M., Zvi, H., Levy, M., Berger, A., and Eidelman, A. The uniqueness of mother-own-infant interactions. *Infant Behavior and Development* 18: 247–252, 1995.

Klaus, M. H. and Kennell, J. H., and Klaus, P. H. *Bonding: Building the foundations of secure attachment and independence.* Cambridge, Mass.: Perseus Books, 1995.

Parke, R. D. *Fatherhood.* Cambridge, Mass.: Harvard University Press, 1996.

Robertson, J., and Robertson, J. Young children in brief separation: A fresh look. *Psychoanalytic Study of the Child* 26: 264–315, 1971.

Rodholm, M., and Larsson, K. Father-infant interaction at the first contact after delivery. *Early Human Development* 3: 21–27, 1979.

Stern, D. *Diary of a baby.* New York: Basic Books, 1990.

Winnicott, D. W. The child, the family, and the outside world. Cambridge, Mass.: Perseus Books, 1987.

——. *Collected Papers: Through pediatrics to psychoanalysis.* New York: Basic Books, 1958.

INDEX

ABOUT THE AUTHORS

Marshall H. Klaus, M.D., internationally known neonatologist and researcher, is the author or coauthor of several standard works in the field, including *Bonding, Care of the High-Risk Newborn,* and *Mothering the Mother,* and an editor of the *Yearbook of Neonatal and Perinatal Medicine.* He teaches pediatrics at the University of California, San Francisco, School of Medicine.

Phyllis H. Klaus, C.S.W., M.F.C.C., teaches and practices psychotherapy at the Erikson Institute in Santa Rosa and practices in Berkeley, California, working especially with the concerns of pregnancy, birth, and the postpartum period. She is coauthor of *Mothering the Mother* and *Bonding.*